Table of Contents

Table of Contents

Introduction

With the dawn of the green revolution and advancements in science and agriculture, human beings shifted from a hunter-gatherer lifestyle toward living comparatively sedentary lives and consuming more processed foods and whole grains instead of proteins and fats. Since it wasn't necessary to hunt for meat any longer, this led to the increase in consumption of complex carbohydrates and sugars, which is not what the body is designed for as per evolution.

The consumption of sugars and carbohydrates is not healthy for the body and can lead to health complications and other issues. If you are looking to lead a life that is devoid of chronic ailments, inflammation, and arthritis, the ketogenic diet is the best way to achieve that. It helps the body get rid of unwanted inflammation, aids weight loss, and increases the body's energy levels throughout the day. The ketogenic diet can help you become healthier and more productive.

The keto diet or the ketogenic diet is a low-carbohydrate, high-fat diet. It is like other low-carbohydrate diets such as the Paleo diet and the Atkins diet. When you increase your consumption of fat and reduce the consumption of carbohydrates, it puts your body into a ketosis state where the body starts burning a lot of fats for meeting the body's energy requirements. The keto diet is well known among weight-loss enthusiasts and fitness communities.

Over 20 different research studies have conclusively proved that the ketogenic diet promotes weight loss and improves your overall health. The ketogenic diet has also shown positive benefits for people suffering from different diseases such as diabetes, cancer, epilepsy, and chronic inflammation. The consumption of large amounts of carbohydrates has been closely linked to inflammation and other ailments.

Carbohydrates are directly broken down into glucose. Moderate amounts of proteins can also be converted to blood sugar. Keto diet is high in fat content. The fats are broken down into ketones by the liver, which then provides energy for different bodily processes, especially for neurological functions. In a state of ketosis, the body (the liver) becomes extremely efficient at burning fat molecules to produce usable energy. The conversion of fats to ketones by the liver is a completely different process, and most of the energy produced in the form of ketones is used by the brain instead of other biological systems. This process is known as ketosis and it is where the diet gets its name.

You will learn all this and more in the course of this book. You will also be introduced to some lip smacking delicious yet healthy ketogenic recipes. So, without any further ado, let us get started.

Chapter One: History of The Ketogenic Diet

The ketogenic diet has been a part of the mainstream dietary practices that were first developed by nutritionists and scientists to be used for controlling seizures in patients that were suffering from epilepsy while removing the limitations of non-mainstream dietary practices such as fasting. Most patients who are suffering from epilepsy can effectively control their seizures by altering their diets without having to use many pharmaceutical medications. It was first popularized during the 1920s and 1930s but was later abandoned in favor of newer pharmaceuticals and anticonvulsant drugs. However, there are some patients (20%-30%) who are still unable to control their seizures despite using different drugs and medications. For these people, the ketogenic diet proved to be very effective and played a very important role in epilepsy management.

The history of the actual ketogenic diet, as we know it today began in 1923 at the Mayo Clinic, with Dr. Russell Wilder at the helm of it. He was the first person who designed what we now know as the classic ketogenic diet. The classic ketogenic diet comprised of four parts of fat for every single part of protein and carbohydrate. The modern keto diet is based on this four-to-one ratio that was developed by Dr. Russell Wilder. However, the early medical practitioners of ancient Greece were already treating diseases such as epilepsy by altering the diet of the patients.

The ketogenic diet achieved mainstream attention and international media exposure during the 1990s when prominent Hollywood celebrities and influencers began promoting the keto diet for controlling and managing epilepsy. Fasting has played a very important role in the treatment of various diseases afflicting mankind for thousands of years and was studied extensively by ancient Indian and Greek philosophers. Hippocratic Corpus described the role that different alterations in diet played in treating and managing epilepsy. In his collection "Epidemics," he also described an account of how a man who had epilepsy was completely cured when he completely abstained from eating certain foods or drinking specific beverages.

Modern scientific studies were also conducted to explore fasting as a potential cure for epilepsy and seizures in France in 1911. At the time, potassium bromide was a popular medication for treating epilepsy, but it was also known for causing a slowdown of the person's mental faculties. However, a trial was conducted where twenty patients who have epilepsy started following a low-calorie vegan diet combined with different fasting regimes. Two of the twenty patients started showing significant improvements; coincidentally, they were the ones who could properly adhere to the prescribed dietary restrictions. Compared to the effects of potassium bromide, the dietary practice was found to reduce the symptoms without affecting the patient's mental abilities.

During the early 20th century, an American nutritionist Bernard Macfadden popularized the practice of fasting as a means of improving general health. Hugh Conklin, who was a student osteopath, popularized fasting as a treatment for managing epilepsy. He proposed that a toxin that was secreted in the intestine was responsible for causing epileptic seizures among epilepsy seizures. He suggested that fasting for a few days would cause the toxin to break down and dissipate. He introduced some epileptic patients to the "water diet," which reportedly cured 50% of the adult patients and 90% of the children.

The fasting theory became more popular due to this, and it was soon adopted as a mainstream treatment method for epilepsy and epileptic seizures. In 1916, it was reported in the New York Medical Journal that Dr. McMurray treated a group of epileptic patients by prescribing them a starch and sugar-free diet coupled with fasting for four years.

Rolling Woodyatt was the first endocrinologist who identified that three water-soluble compounds were produced by the liver due to a result of fasting or a high-fat low-carbohydrate diet. These compounds were acetone, acetoacetate, and β-hydroxybutyrate, collectively known as ketones or ketone bodies. Dr. Russell Wilder of the Mayo Clinic was the first to classify this dietary practice as the "ketogenic diet" and promoted its use as a treatment for epilepsy.

Later, further research was conducted during the 1960s, which showed that the consumption of MCTs or medium-chain triglycerides (complex fats) produced more ketones per unit of energy. This was because these MCTs are quickly transported to the liver through the hepatic portal vein instead of the lymphatic pathways. Peter Huttenlocher developed a ketogenic diet in which 60% of the calories were derived from different MCT oils. These allowed more proteins and carbohydrates to be included into the ketogenic diet as compared to the classic ketogenic diet. This meant that the diet could be made more appealing and enjoyable for children by adding more carbohydrates and proteins.

Chapter Two: The Science Behind Ketogenic Diet

Mainstream media has been abuzz with different anecdotes and accounts of the amazing benefits that a ketogenic diet can have on your health. You might have noticed that every year is marked by the rise in popularity of a new diet fad followed by a subsequent decline. Most of this is possible due to the figurative echo chamber created by the Internet and social media websites, but there is no actual evidence to commend these diet fads. However, the ketogenic diet is not one of these diet fads, because there is actual science behind how it works, supported by years of extensive research scientific studies.

The ketogenic diet is centered on the different ketones or ketone bodies, which are complex molecules that act as the body's natural energy supply in addition to the brain. The ketones are specifically used by the brain to satisfy its massive energy requirements. It is important to know that the brain is the organ with one of the highest work rates and accounts for the consumption of 20% of the total energy produced by the body in the form of glucose, ketones, and ATP (Adenosine Triphosphates) which are the three basic energy currencies of the body. The gist of the ketogenic diet is that it is supposed to put your body into a state of "ketosis" or "ketogenesis," where it's capacity to burn fat as an energy supply increases significantly, instead of solely relying on glucose. So, what exactly is ketosis?

Here's the deal, "ketosis" refers to "generating ketones." The major source of ketones is fats and triglycerides. This means that to stimulate your body to enter a state of ketosis, your body will have to start deriving energy from fats instead of carbohydrates. Ketogenic diet help you naturally hack your body into a state of starvation where it begins burning its fat reserves, which is like what happens in fasting.

You will have to reduce your daily carbohydrate consumption drastically. Most people follow a staple diet that is very high in carb content in the form of processed grain, whole grains, corn, and derived products, flour and flour-based products, and sugar-based products. The daily consumption of carbs can exceed 100 grams a day for most individuals who follow these "normal" diets.

When your diet is heavily based on carbohydrates instead of fats and healthy proteins, your liver will store these carbohydrates in a comparatively simple storage mechanism in the form of fats or break down the simpler carbohydrates into glucose, which acts as an energy supply. However, when you start following a ketogenic diet that is high in fat content and low in carbohydrates, interesting changes start happening in your body's metabolism. An adult human brain normally runs on 100 grams of glucose per day. However, when your diet is low in carbohydrates and sugars, your liver is unable to produce enough glucose to supply the body's energy requirements. This is when it begins to produce ketones or ketone bodies to provide energy for the body and the brain. It is perfectly healthy and natural for the brain to function on ketones, and this process gradually increases from 0% to 70% in three weeks. What is even more interesting is that during these three weeks, your somatic tissues (other bodily tissues excluding the nervous system and brain) begin to use mostly fats and free fatty acids (produced from the breakdown of stored fats) as a source of energy.

In a state of ketosis, the liver is breaking down fats into ketones at a very high rate. The concentration of acetone, acetoacetate, and beta-hydroxybutyrate increases in the blood. Some of these molecules are excreted through sweat molecules, breath, and urine during the initial stages. Most of the acetoacetate and beta-hydroxybutyrate molecules are sent to different tissues of the body to provide energy.

Ketones vs. Glucose as An Energy Source

In a non-ketosis state, carbohydrates are broken down into glucose or stored as fats. The glucose is transported through the bloodstream to the different cells and tissues. The glucose is then converted into pyruvate, which then enters the Citric Acid Cycle, where it generates energy in the form of Adenosine Triphosphate (ATP). Although all this may sound like a scientific banter, the process is a significant metabolic activity that generates energy and keeps us alive. The whole process of ATP production is an important metabolic process that provides energy to the body.

Now, when there is insufficient glucose in the body to generate ATP from the pyruvate and supply energy, then the body starts deriving energy from fatty acids. This is known as ketosis. The process of ketosis not only produces ketones but also produces a good amount of ATP too. You do not necessarily need to starve your body to induce a state of ketosis. The only thing that you need is to remove carbohydrates from your diet. This not only includes refined carbohydrates such as sugars, sucrose, and high fructose corn syrup but complex carbohydrates such as starches and glutens too. Once the body has no source of carbohydrates and, consequently, glucose, it is forced to enter a state of ketosis because the brain needs some form of energy in the form of glucose or ketones to keep the body alive. So, the increased consumption of fats and proteins will not lead to excessive weight gain or obesity because they are broken down into ketones by the liver to keep your body going.

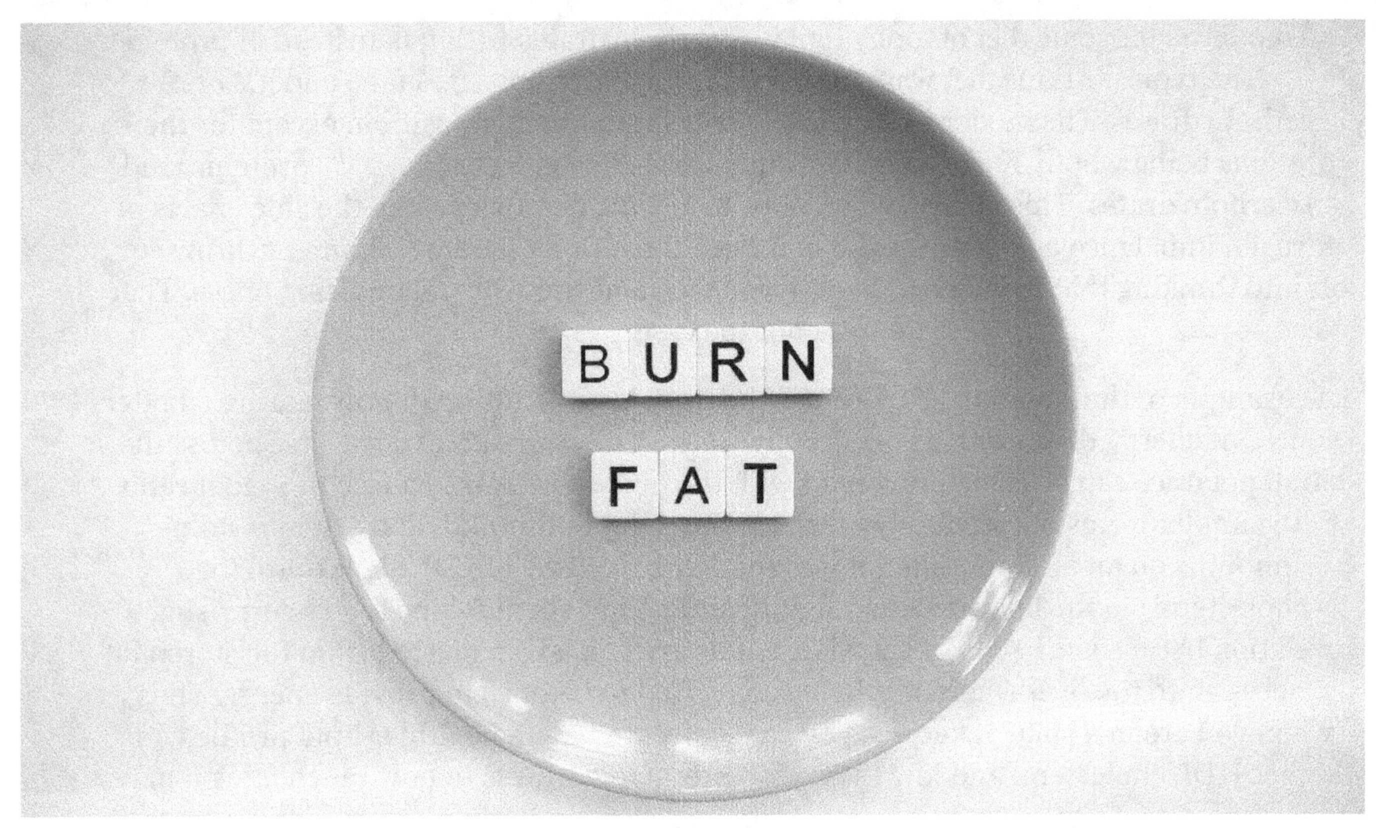

The Atkins Diet vs. Ketogenic Diet

The Atkins diet rose to prominence several years, and many people reported to have lost significant weight after following the diet regime. The Atkins diet is very similar to the ketogenic diet as it also removes carbohydrates from the diet and replaces it with proteins. The most common thing that was reported by several people following the Atkins diet was that they felt much less hungry than compared to when they were following their previous diet. This suggests that the calories that were being derived from proteins satisfied your energy requirement for a longer period as compared to most carb-based diets. The feeling of being full was what translated to people willingly eating lesser portions of food and achieving

weight loss. However, the Atkins diet also has its share of cons and side effects. The excessive quantities of protein could have a serious impact on the nitrogen balance of the body and

health complications. A high risk of dehydration is there that is associated with the Atkins diet, and over prolonged periods, there can be the formation of kidney stones due to the excessive levels of nitrogen and urea in the body.

The modern ketogenic diet of today replaces carbohydrates with fats instead of proteins. The typical Atkins diet was comprised of 75% proteins, 25% fats, and 5% of carbohydrates. The modern ketogenic diet is similar in composition, except for the proteins being wholly replaced by fats and vice versa, i.e., 75% fats, 25% proteins, and 5% carbohydrates. This allows the modern ketogenic diet to sidestep the side effects of nitrogen imbalance and other health complications. Don't let the fat content throw you off into thinking that it will be unhealthy for you, and you will end up being obese. That is not the case.

The example of the Antarctic explorers is the best demonstration of how fats are a better source of energy than proteins or carbohydrates. They were able to traverse across the harsh polar ice cap by consuming food with the highest possible calorie to weight ratio. In simpler terms, it essentially meant nothing but butter and fats. After spending months on an all-butter diet, it was seen that the level of LDL cholesterol (bad cholesterol) in the body declined significantly. That shouldn't be a very surprising revelation because in a state of ketosis, the fats are being transported from the stored fat reserves into the liver where it is being converted to ketones to provide energy. Thus, when you are in a state of ketosis, you can expect to have a healthier lipid profile with higher HDL cholesterol and low LWD cholesterol, regardless of how much fat you may be eating.

Chapter Three: Losing Fat on A Ketogenic Diet

As mentioned earlier, you begin to lose fat when following a ketogenic diet in the same way that most diets work: your body begins to burn the stored fat reserves instead of accumulating fat into them. However, this mechanism is not entirely straightforward and not as simple as "counting calories." Since everybody type responds differently to different types of calories, for example, one hundred calories of spinach are different from one hundred calories of ice cream.

The most important factor that aids in weight loss is that the ketogenic diet reduces your hunger drastically, which consequently forces more fat to come out of the storage reserves and used for energy. The fats are being forced out instead of being stored inside. The ketogenic diet is also responsible for regulating insulin levels, which makes it easier for your body to take advantage of leptin-induced satiety.

When the insulin levels are relatively low daily, fat is constantly being extracted from the stored fat reserves, and the process ramps and happens more readily as the body becomes used to burning fats for energy instead of carbohydrates. The ketogenic diet can also help you wean yourself off the dopamine addiction, which can be accompanying spiking blood sugar levels.

As mentioned earlier, this plays a very important role in raising HDL cholesterol levels and lowering LDL cholesterol levels and triglyceride levels in patients suffering from obesity. The human body is designed to run more efficiently by burning fats instead of carbohydrates, and this is supported by the evidence provided by ancient history and evolutionary biology.

Chapter Four: Pros of The Ketogenic Diet

The ketogenic diet has a similar objective to most dietary regimes, promoting fat loss and improving general health and fitness levels. However, there are both benefits and side effects associated with following this diet and having a good knowledge of these effects is essential in practicing the ketogenic diet successfully with the best possible results. The ketogenic diet has several benefits, and the pros clearly outweigh the cons, but you should have a good knowledge of the possible side effects so that you can sidestep them.

Let us first look at the positive health benefits that the ketogenic diet provides for the human body:

Improved Memory and Cognition

As we learned earlier, ketogenic diet were first used at the Mayo Clinic in the early 1920s for treating children who were suffering from epilepsy. Although the exact mechanism behind seizure prevention and epilepsy control due to the ketogenic diet is still a medical mystery, some scientists believe that the phenomenon has something to do with increased stability of neurons and axons of the central nervous system and the proliferation and development of mitochondrial cells in the brain and other mitochondrial enzymes.

The mitochondria are present in the cells, and they are known as the "powerhouse" of the cells. These are the sites where glucose or ketone is broken down into Adenosine Triphosphate in the presence of oxygen and water. These are the furnaces that burn fuel to produce energy that the body utilizes to keep you going every day. This means that the more mitochondria your cells possess, the more efficient they are at producing energy and carrying out their respective functions. The human brain prefers ketones as a better energy source as compared to glucose, but due to modern carb-based diets that comprise of processed foods and sugars, our body is compelled to use glucose as an alternative energy source. This works too, but it isn't as efficient and effective as ketones and ketone bodies.

Another research study has also given some serious attention to the ketogenic diet and Alzheimer's disease. It was discovered that adults with impaired mental faculties showed an increase in cognition and enhance memory power when they were put on a strict low-carb ketogenic diet. Another different growing research body also discovered that ketogenic diet showed an improvement in all stages of dementia. Ketosis was also discovered to be effective against Parkinson's disease and other neurodegenerative diseases. Patients suffering from these diseases began showing an improvement in mental clarity and focus and reported less frequent migraines and seizures. These effects are also related to increased stability in blood sugar levels and improvement in brain chemistry, which leads to subsequent improvement in brain function, memory, and cognition. Further research is still required to solidify the correlations between keto diet and brain health. However, most of the studies, which we have just discussed, clearly indicate that ketogenic diet provides neuroprotective benefits in some form. A new study has also found that children that were following a ketogenic diet showed increased alertness and higher cognitive functioning.

Prevention of Cancer

An article was published by Doctor Dom D'Agostino's lab in 2015 titled "Ketone supplementation decreases the viability of tumor cells and prolongs the lifespan of mice suffering from metastatic cancer." The article investigated how cancer tissues expressed an abnormal metabolism when there was an increase in the consumption of glucose. This was mainly caused due to genetic mutations and mitochondrial dysfunction within the different issues that were caused by a high carb diet. The article also discussed how unlike the natural cells of the body, cancer tissues are not able to use ketone bodies for energy effectively as compared to glucose or ATP (Adenosine Triphosphate). In addition, the ketones bodies also inhibit the viability and proliferation of cultured tumor cells. In more recent years, this diet has been extensively investigated on how it helps to prevent and treat certain types of cancers. Another study found that the keto diet was found to be complementary to chemotherapy treatment and radiation treatment in people who have cancer. This is because a ketogenic diet increases the oxidative stress in different cancerous tissues and cells compared to the normal somatic cells.

Improving Cardiovascular Health

If you follow the ketogenic diet correctly and healthily, there is strong evidence that suggests that the keto diet can improve cardiovascular health by reducing the level of LDL cholesterol and increasing HDL cholesterol levels. The HDL signifies the "good" cholesterol, which healthy for your body, and the LDL is the "bad" cholesterol, which is associated with most heart diseases.

The ketogenic diet also helps regulate the blood pressure levels and keeps the triglyceride levels in check. Although it may seem counterintuitive that consuming a high percentage of fat as a part of your diet can lower the cholesterol levels, in reality, the consumption of high amount of carbohydrates (especially sugars, sucrose, and fructose syrup) is the major factor that is responsible for increasing the levels of triglycerides and "bad" cholesterol.

Reduces Inflammation

The ketogenic diet is profoundly known for its anti-inflammatory properties and helps provide relief when it comes to a host of other health problems that can be caused by inflammation. What is inflammation? It is the body's natural reaction mechanism when it is subjected to stress beyond a certain limit or is invaded by foreign particles. Contrary to popular belief, it isn't an actual disease but the body's way of retaliating to different diseases. For instance, when you sprain your ankle, you have stressed it beyond its natural limits. The body's natural response to this excessive stress is to cause swelling and tenderness at the site of the sprain. The injury is naturally cushioned by the increased water content, which acts as a protective layer that prevents further aggravation of the injury. You will also observe a change in the skin tone at the site of the injury. This is because lymphocytes and antibodies (white blood cells) localize at the site of the injury to tackle any foreign bacteria or harmful toxins, which could be causing the injury or infection (inflammation is also caused by infections). Inflammation on its own is beneficial for the body and protects it.

So how does the keto diet fit into the picture? That is a common thing to ponder. When you are on a normal carbohydrate-based diet, your body, specifically your liver, is used to converting these carbohydrates into glucose. The glucose is then used to supply energy in the form of ATP to the different parts of the body. Your liver and digestive system do not face any problem when it comes to processing simpler carbohydrates that are found in fruits and vegetables (e.g., glucose, fructose, and sucrose). It is the more complex carbohydrates that cause complications, as the liver is unable to break them down into glucose rapidly.

Complex carbohydrates are mostly found in foods derived from processed grains and whole grains such as pasta, bread, barley, and other baked products. These complex carbohydrates are converted to simpler metabolites first, instead of being directly broken down into glucose molecules. However, your liver is not designed to carry out this process continues, and the metabolites are stored into the fat reserves along with the body's fat cells. These metabolites do not perform any specific function in the metabolic activities and play no role in the body's overall functioning whatsoever. Since the body's natural response to the presence of foreign compounds with no significant role to play is to trigger inflammation, it is exactly what happens. This inflammation can bring about other ailments in the form of chronic pain, arthritis, and skin complications.

When you switch to this diet, your body is constantly burning fats instead of carbs because that is what your diet is mostly composed of. Instead of breaking down complex carbohydrates into harmful inflammation-causing metabolites, the liver is consistently burning free fatty acids extracted from the food you eat your body's stored fat reserves as well. Glycerides or fats have a simpler chemical structure and composition as compared to most carbohydrates; therefore, these molecules are readily broken down by the liver to produce ketones. This sidesteps the body's inflammatory response towards foreign particles and significantly reduces inflammation.

Improved Sleeping Habits and Increased Energy Levels

Although this effect is not instant, by the first week of the keto diet, you may notice an increase in the energy levels and a drastic reduction in the craving for carbohydrates or carb-rich food products. This is because the state of ketosis also stabilizes the levels of insulin (and other hormones) in the bloodstream. The human brain functions at a higher rate when it is functioning on a ketone-based energy supply instead of glucose. Although the actual mechanism behind this is unknown, and there are no concrete reasons for its causation other than an increase in the number of mitochondria, the brain is healthier when your diet is low on carbohydrates. Ketones, in general, tend to be a more effective and efficient source of energy for the human body than glucose. Most people report that they are much more focused and energetic throughout the day when they are on a ketogenic diet.

As for improvements in sleep, it is still not completely proven. A research study showed that the ketogenic diet could improve sleeping patterns by reducing the amount of REM sleep (sleep characterized by Random Eye Movement) and increasing the duration of slow-wave sleep patterns, which subsequently has a positive effect on the circadian rhythms and brain health. While it is still relatively unclear, it is most probably related to the complex shifts in the brain biochemistry caused due to the brain's use of ketones as an energy source supplemented by the fact that the body's fat reserves are constantly being utilized.

Improving Kidney Function

We have already seen that earlier non-conventional dietary practices such as the Atkins's diet were very high in its protein content, which subsequently led to various diseases such as gout, kidney stones, and other nephrology complications. It was also observed that diets that were unnaturally high in protein or carbohydrate content elevated the levels of calcium, oxalate, phosphorus, and uric acid due to the liver's inability to breakdown excessive quantities of carbs and proteins. Instead of helping people, most of the fad diets that momentarily crop up in mainstream media can cause more harm than good in the form of dehydration, obesity, and addiction to complex carbohydrates and saccharides (complex sugars).

The ketogenic diet is the opposite of most diet regimes and contains a high amount of healthy fats instead of proteins and carbohydrates. It is easier for the liver and the digestive system to process these fats instead of conventional proteins and carbohydrates, which also happens to be the reason behind all the health complications. However, there is something important to notice here; the ketogenic diet also increases the levels of uric acid and urea in the body, but it is temporary and usually comes down over time. Drinking enough amounts of water and staying hydrated will help you achieve that. Just in case one may panic, the level of uric acid will promptly increase in roughly the same time frame required by the body to increase its production of ketones. However, this effect is short-lived, and after a month or six weeks, the level uric acid decreases and establishes a normal level. Ketosis will not cause the formation of any kidney stones or other urinary complications if you supplement it with adequate consumption of water and physical activity.

Improves Gastrointestinal Health

As we have already seen, grain-based carbohydrate-rich foods and nightshade vegetables such as tomatoes and potatoes can increase the tendency of acid reflux and other gastrointestinal issues such as heartburn and indigestion. As discussed in earlier chapters, the liver and the digestive system has trouble processing and breaking down higher complex carbohydrates. Food and beverages high quantities of carbohydrates or complex sugars are not healthy for your body because of this very reason. If you are eating lots of pasta, sourdough bread, or drinking vast quantities of soda-based beverages such as Coca Cola and milkshakes, your body will probably function at a lower level of efficacy, and you will generally feel tired and lethargic throughout the day because of your poor dietary practices.

Research studies have also shown that diets containing high amounts of carbohydrates or proteins can cause the formation of stones in the gall bladder. Although it is very important to note that if you can correctly supplement a high protein diet with adequate hydration and physical exercise, you will observe some positive changes in your health. However, this is not the case usually, and a high protein or high carbohydrate diet can overwork the gall bladder. This leads to calcification of different minerals and salts in the gall bladder, which consequently leads to the formation of gall bladder stones. If your diet is high in fat content instead of carbohydrates or proteins, it aids the functioning of the gall bladder and helps clear out the residue and keep things functioning smoothly, preventing the formation of gall bladder stones.

Improved Female Reproductive Health

An extensive research journal published in 2013 highlighted the evidence of ketogenic diet improving fertility and reproductive health in females. Some clinical studies also showed that ketogenic diet was effective in treating PCOS or Polycystic Ovary Syndrome, and a low carb diet can reduce or even eliminate other symptoms of reproductive disorders such as menstrual cramps, irregular periods, acne and abnormal weight gain.

Hormones play an important role in the ovarian cycle of the female reproductive system. When you are in a constant state of ketosis, your body can regulate glucose and ketone levels in the blood effectively. This can significantly improve the endocrine system efficiency, which is solely responsible for the regulation of hormone secretions and the functions that these hormones are associated with. The level of hormones, such as insulin, oxytocin, and estrogen, are stabilized, and this helps regulate the ovarian cycle much more efficiently. Since the state of ketosis also improves the production and utilization of energy in the body, it reduces the symptoms of menstrual complications such as irregular discharge, low fertility, and pain.

Improved Eyesight

This is one of the indirect benefits that the ketogenic provides. Although an improvement in vision and eyesight is not due to the direct influence of the process of ketosis, ketogenic diet helps the body regulate the level of glucose (blood sugar). Any patient who has diabetes will tell you that this has a drastically detrimental effect on the eyes, and it can also increase the risk of forming cataracts.

What ketosis does is shift the body's energy supply from glucose to ketones. This means that your body has a higher concentration of ketones, fueling it instead of glucose, and this effectively reduces blood sugar levels. This reduces the tendency of cataract formation and improves eyesight and general vision health.

Increase in Muscle Mass and Endurance

In the first chapter, we discussed the process of ketosis and how it increases the production of ketones or ketone bodies. The three types of ketones that are produced by the liver are acetone, acetoacetate, and beta-hydroxybutyrate (BHB). These ketones provide energy to the different parts of the body. Acetone and acetoacetate are primarily involved in supplying energy for the brain and different neurological processes. However, beta-hydroxybutyrate has been shown to promote the formation of muscle tissues. Although most of this evidence is anecdotal, there are hundreds of bodybuilders and fitness experts who use and promote a ketogenic approach to gaining muscle mass and reduce the formation of fat reserves in the body.

Endurance is something that is more commonly associated with triathletes and other ultra-endurance athletes. This does not mean that it does not concern other average human beings. Endurance is the ability of your body to maintain a steady level of energy production and work output rate for a prolonged period. It translates to your body's stamina and the capacity to efficiently use energy. There are a handful of research studies that provide direct evidence indicating that the energy derived from a unit quantity of free fatty acid is much more than that from the same quantity of glucose (derived from simple carbohydrates, proteins or sugars).

In short, when your body is in a state of ketosis, you can function more efficiently, translating to improved mental and physical performance. Although "carbo-loading" was a very common practice among athletes where they were consuming large quantities of carb-rich foods such as pasta and bread, these concepts have been rapidly debunked and discredited in recent years. Every endurance athlete will tell you that it is easier to improve physical performance by following a ketogenic diet instead of a traditional carbohydrate-rich diet.

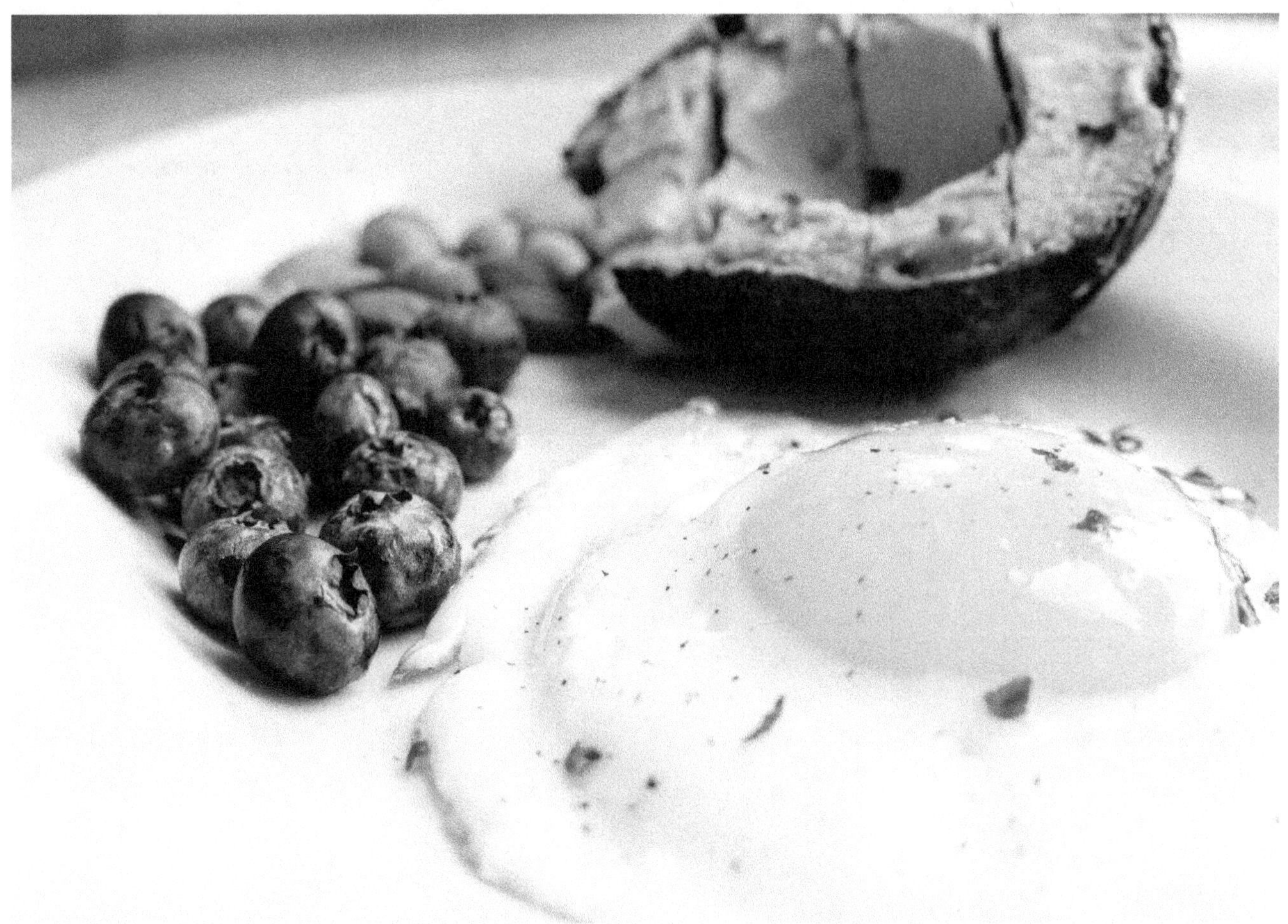

Chapter Five: Side Effects Associated with Ketogenic diet

It seems like we have been praising the positive effects of ketosis and the ketogenic diet for too long. However, if you are planning to follow the ketogenic regime, it is important that you are aware of the possible side effects that accompany a keto lifestyle. In consideration, these side effects are nothing compared to the adverse effects that are associated with anticonvulsant medications, which are commonly used for treating diseases such as epilepsy and epileptic seizures. Let us take a closer look at some of these potential side effects.

Keto Flu

The keto flu is very popular among keto enthusiasts. This is very commonly observed during the initial stages of ketosis. It is mainly caused as a result of the body entering a low carbohydrate state. Since your body is habituated to using carbohydrates for deriving energy, a sudden shift towards free fatty acids as an energy source can cause the keto flu. When you are in a state of ketosis, your body is forced to burn ketones to derive energy instead of using glucose. However, this shift of energy source can be manifested as a feeling that is not very pleasant and comfortable. This is what the keto flu is; it is not caused due to a viral or bacterial infection.

The keto flu symptoms can be different depending on one individual to another. It may include everything from weakness and irritability to constipation, vomiting, nausea, and headaches. When your body is initially subjected to a change in energy source from burning sugars to burning the body's stored fat reserves, it increases ketone production. The ketones are frequently expelled from the body through frequent urination and increased sweating. This often leads to dehydration and symptoms that are very common with flu, such as dizziness, fatigue, nausea, vomiting, and soreness of the muscles.

The frequent urination and loss of water can lead to an inevitable loss of electrolytes, which can further exacerbate these symptoms. Since your body is previously used to consuming carbohydrates as a source of energy, it can cause intense sugar cravings, loss of attention/focus, and brain fog in the initial stage of ketosis, which also accounts for the symptoms of keto flu. You can sidestep this by making sure that you stay hydrated throughout the day and subject yourself to adequate physical activity. The keto flu will only last for a week or so, and you will begin to feel the positive effects of ketosis very soon.

Kidney and Heart Damage

The body is low on essential electrolytes and nutrients during the initial stages of ketosis due to constant urination and dehydration. This means that your body is low on important electrolytes such as potassium, magnesium, and sodium, which are responsible for regulating different cardiovascular and renal functions. This can increase the risk of developing kidney damage and kidney failure in extreme cases. Dehydration is the major driving factor in causing kidney failure and kidney stones.

The cardiovascular functions of the hearts and its rhythmic beating (systole and diastole) are essential for maintaining the beating of the heart. The deficiency of sodium and potassium can cause severe arrhythmia and cardiovascular diseases.

Yo-Yo Dieting

This is a case of a lack of control and self-discipline instead of a direct side effect of ketogenic diet. Many people have great difficulty in consistently following a restrictive diet on a permanent basis. An undetermined individual may succumb to the intense sugar craving or carbohydrate cravings that accompany the initial stages of ketosis. This constant to-and-fro shift between a normal diet and a ketogenic diet can have an overall negative effect on the body. The change in diet from carbohydrates to fats and vice versa can cause an abnormal increase in body weight and increases the risk of mortality.

Nutritional Concerns

There is a common fear among some nutritionists and health experts of the potential long-term negative effects that are associated with a high intake of unhealthy fats. The keto diet is centered on fats, and they can be very low on certain vegetables, fruits, whole grains, and legumes. Although the ketogenic diet and ketosis, in general, can be healthy in many aspects, the diet also tends to miss out on some essential nutrients such as fibers (roughage), minerals, vitamins, and phytochemicals (chemicals derived from plants). This can have a significant impact on human health over the long term, and it is manifested as a loss of bone density and an increased risk of contracting chronic diseases.

We all know the importance of vegetables, and there are many studies that conclusively prove the significant positive effects of whole plant foods. These include a reduced risk of diseases such as osteoporosis, cardiovascular diseases, type-2 diabetes, and cancer. The positive effects that you may experience after following a ketogenic diet are important, but it does not mean that vegetables are irrelevant. You need to periodically supplement your keto diet with some vegetables and fruits in order to maintain optimal health.

Short Term Side Effects

There are numerous short-term side effects that are experienced in the early stages of ketosis, more particularly when they begin their keto diet with an initial period of fasting. Some of these side effects are:

- Hypoglycemia.

- Frequent urination.

- Increased Hunger.

- Fatigue.

- Tachycardia.

- Sweating and chills.

- Anxiety and irritability.

- Loss of focus.

- Nausea.

- Constipations

- Low-grade acidosis.

These side effects are usually short-lived and subside as the body gradually adapts to the new keto diet, and it becomes a state of normalcy.

Chapter Six: Impact of Ketogenic Diet on Insulin

Insulin is one of the major hormonal secretions produced by the body's endocrine system. Its primary function is metabolizing the carbohydrates that you consume in your diet. Insulin is not necessarily bad, but it can be a hindrance when it comes to achieving certain health-related objectives. If your main objective is getting your body into a state of stable ketosis, insulin is your enemy. However, if you are looking to bulk up and gain muscle mass, insulin is the best thing that could happen to you.

The whole point of following a ketogenic diet is forcing your body to enter a state of ketosis where it produces ketones for providing energy in contrary to glucose or carbohydrates. This is the real essence of the ketogenic diet and the thing that makes it work. Insulin hinders the process of ketosis and suppresses the production of ketones in the liver.

If you want your body to enter a state of ketosis and maintain it in that state, you need to minimize the production of insulin as much as possible. The easiest way to stimulate this change is by altering your diet and what you eat daily. The production of insulin is triggered by the consumption of certain foods, and changing your diet effectively alters the production of insulin. This is what the ketogenic diet does. The ketogenic diet aims at minimizing the production of insulin by reducing the intake of carbohydrates and proteins. The diet keeps the level of carbohydrates and proteins as low as possible without causing any health issues.

Chapter Seven: Ketogenic Diet and Menstruation

Although there is a good number of people who believe that the keto diet can significantly improve health by regulating cholesterol levels and inducing weight loss, a sudden reduction in the consumption of carbohydrates, which is encouraged by the ketogenic diet place, can have a significant impact on the body. A female's menstrual cycle is one of these important health parameters that can be affected by this sudden diet change. The sudden lack of certain nutrients that foods can provide can affect the menstrual cycle in negative ways.

Crystal C. Karges, a dietician, believes that cutting out a major macronutrient that your body is accustomed to receiving can create gaps in a woman's nutrition and alter her general biochemistry. There are several other experts who have investigated the subject of how the keto diet can affect your periods and menstrual cycles. We will be looking into a few salient points that these experts recommend keeping in mind if you are considering going keto.

The lack of carbohydrates in your diet can cause issues with menstruation and ovulation. Carbohydrates act as a primary source of energy, and the body becomes accustomed to processing the carbs that are consumed every day. When the consumption of carbohydrates is promptly reduced on a drastic scale, it alters the metabolism of the body. The liver and the endocrine system, which is accustomed to processing carbs and using glucose to derive energy, goes haywire when you start eating food that is high in fats and low in carbohydrates. This can cause fluctuations of hormones and can mess with menstrual cycles and ovulation.

When you initially begin following a ketogenic diet, your body's supply of calories cuts down promptly, and this can cause irregular periods. It has been observed that irregular periods or amenorrhea is caused by stress. Amenorrhea is a reproductive complication where there is an absence of menstruation for a period of three months or more. Stress, coupled with low carb diet and calorific restrictions and physical stress, can induce irregular periods. Since most people (females and males) decide to follow the ketogenic diet with ambitions of weight loss, this drastic drop of calories, along with physical stress and periods of fasting, can disrupt the cycle of periods in the female reproductive system.

The ketogenic diet forces the body into a state of ketosis. An important thing to note is that ketogenesis is marked by a fluctuation in the secretion of different hormones of the endocrine system. The menstrual cycle is regulated by different hormones, such as leptin, oxytocin, and estrogen. These hormones are crucially involved in the menstrual process and need to be at certain levels for different stages of the menstrual cycle to commence and end properly. Leptin is a hormone that is very important for having normal periods.

Ketosis can lead to rapid weight loss. Many research studies have shown that rapidly losing a lot of pounds in a short time period can lead to sharp drops in the secretion of estrogen. Estrogen, as we already know, plays a very important role in menstruation, and fluctuations in its levels can cause adverse and unwanted changes in the menstrual cycles. In simpler words, too much weight loss can mess up the menstrual cycle.

Considering what we have just seen, it is important to consult a physician before taking part in any rigorous diet plan so that you do not face any problems related to reproductive health. If you already have a doctor, he will be familiar with your complete medical history and overall health parameters and tendencies. This can be very helpful in evading the adverse effects that diet plans, such as the ketogenic diet have on female reproductive health.

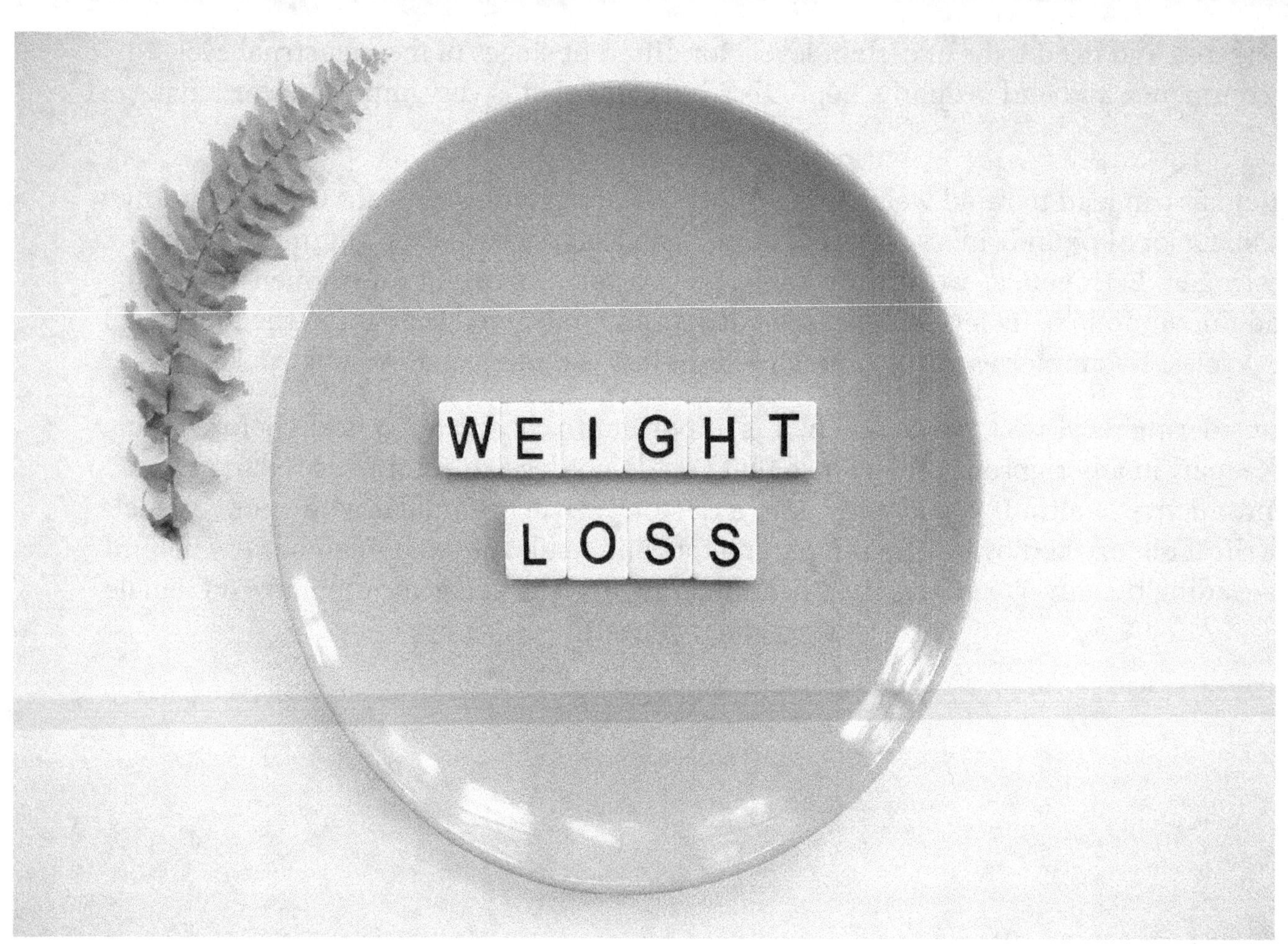
WEIGHT
LOSS

Chapter Eight: Practicing the Ketogenic Diet

Now that we have seen the positive, as well as the negative effects of keto diet and ketosis on the body, let us delve into how you can begin your keto journey. We know that the keto diet is based on increasing fat intake and drastically reducing the number of carbohydrates in your diet. There are three basic types of ketogenic diet:

Standard Ketogenic Diet (SKD)

The standard ketogenic diet consists of a very low amount of carbohydrates and high-fat content. 75% of fats, 20% proteins, and 5% carbohydrates form the SKD.

Cyclical Ketogenic Diet (CKD)

The cyclic ketogenic diet incorporates periods of comparatively higher carbo refeeds. It usually follows five ketogenic days, followed by two high-carb days or "cheat days."

Targeted Ketogenic Diet (SKD)

This TKD diet is like the standard ketogenic diet barring the fact that you can add carbohydrates to your diet before or after workouts.

High Protein Ketogenic Diet

This diet is also very similar to the standard ketogenic diet but includes a higher content of protein. 60% of fats, 35% proteins, and 5% carbohydrates make a high protein ketogenic diet.

What Should You Eat?

Here is an exhaustive list of foods that you should be incorporating into your keto diet:

- Meats such as red meats in the form of steaks, sausages, bacon, and ham.

- Eggs, preferably omega—3 whole eggs.

- Butter and cream from grass-fed sources.

- Unprocessed cheese such as cheddar, mozzarella, blue cheese, and goat cheese.

- Avocado and avocado oils.

- Nuts and dry fruits such as walnuts, almonds, chia seeds, flax seeds, and pumpkin seeds.

- Healthy oils like coconut oil and virgin olive oil.

- Fatty fish like mackerel, salmon, tuna, and trout.

What Should You Avoid Eating?

Ketogenic diet focuses on reducing the consumption of high carb foods. Here is a list of foods that you should try avoiding or eliminating from your diet plan.

- Sugars and products containing fructose corn syrup such as fruit juice, smoothies, sodas, ice creams, cakes, and sweets should be reduced.

- Whole grains and processed grains that contain a lot of starch are a source of unwanted complex carbohydrates. You should reduce your intake of wheat-based products such as cereal, rice, and pasta.

- Fruits are supposed to be very healthy, but not all of them are beneficial when you are trying to go keto. Reduce the consumption of fruits, but you should still have small portions of berries and apples from time to time.

- Beans and legumes like kidney beans, lentils, peas, and chickpeas are rich in carbohydrates, which is counterproductive for ketosis. Avoid eating these too often.

- Tubers and root vegetables like carrots, sweet potatoes, potatoes, and parsnips are rich in starch, which can hinder ketosis.

- Processed foods such as packaged products are high in carbs and additives/preservatives. You can improve ketosis by eliminating them from your diet.

- Unhealthy fats are common in most cuisines. Inferior vegetable oils and mayonnaise are some examples of unhealthy fats that you should be avoiding while going keto.

- Alcoholic beverages such as beer and vodka contain hoops and glutens, which are forms of carbohydrates. Having a drink can remove your body from ketosis.

- Diet foods such as "sugar-free" sweets and Diet Coke contain large amounts of sugar alcohols instead of conventional sugar-based foods. This can affect the production of ketones and reduce ketosis in some cases.

A Sample Ketogenic Diet Plan for The Week

To make things easier, we have a sample ketogenic diet meal plan for the first week of your keto journey. You can follow this regime to try your hand at ketosis and see how your body responds to the ketogenic diet.

MONDAY

Breakfast: Bacon with eggs and tomatoes.

Lunch: Almond mild with peanut butter or cocoa powder or a Stevia milkshake

Dinner: Meatloaf with Parmesan, broccoli, and a light salad.

TUESDAY

Breakfast: A ketogenic milkshake.

Lunch: Chicken salad with a dressing of olive oil and feta cheese.

Dinner: Meatballs with vegetables and cheddar cheese.

WEDNESDAY

Breakfast: Eggs with tomatoes and basil or a goat cheese omelet.

Lunch: Shrimp salad with avocadoes and an olive oil dressing

Dinner: Salmon with asparagus and coconut butter.

THURSDAY

Breakfast: A ham and cheese omelet with steamed greens.

Lunch: Stir-fried beef cooked with vegetables in coconut oil

Dinner: Chicken salad with a dressing of cream cheese and pesto with some vegetables.

FRIDAY

Breakfast: Sugar-free yogurt with cocoa powder, stevia, or peanut butter.

Lunch: Ham and cheese sandwiches with some dry fruits.

Dinner: Bacon with eggs and cheese.

SATURDAY

Breakfast: Omelet of avocado, peppers, onions, spices accompanied with salsa.

Lunch: A bun-less burger with a side of guacamole, salsa or cheese

Dinner: Steak and eggs with a salad.

SUNDAY

Breakfast: Fried eggs with mushrooms and bacon.

Lunch: Dry fruits and celery sticks accompanied with salsa or guacamole.

Dinner: Fish, eggs, and spinach.

Chapter Nine: Mistakes to Avoid While on Ketogenic Diet

Due to a lack of research and database of information when it comes to the ketogenic diet, it can be difficult to gauge your progress. Your ambitions might be focused on losing weight or gaining muscle mass; whatever be the case, what is certain is that the keto diet is a restrictive diet plan, and it can be tough to follow it consistently and correctly. To ensure that you get the best out of your ketogenic lifestyle, you should avoid these mistakes.

Increasing Your Fat Consumption Too Quickly

Before you caught the keto diet, you might have spent years eating cereals for breakfasts, sandwiches for lunch and pasta for dinner. In simpler words, your body has been accustomed to eating and processing high carb foods. After getting on the keto train, you might want to go hard and reduce your consumption of carbohydrates to less than 20 grams per day. This is a drastic change for your body and can make it go haywire. The correct way is to ease your body into ketosis instead of shocking it by abruptly changing everything that it is usually accustomed to. It is safer to taper down your carbohydrate consumption instead of cutting it off suddenly.

Dehydration

It is easy to forget about your intake of water when you are completely immersed in controlling your portions of food. However, it is important to remember to take frequent sips from your water bottle throughout the day while your body is in a state of ketosis. Dehydration is a common thing that most keto enthusiasts suffer from without even noticing it. While following a ketogenic diet, you are completely changing your body's energy supply from carbs to fats. This can cause fluctuations in the levels of different bodily fluids and disrupt the electrolytic balance. Also, most of the carbs that might have been stored in the body are gradually depleted in the state of ketosis. This process involves the loss of water, which causes dehydration.

We have also seen how the body's production of ketone ramps up in the initial stage of ketosis. These ketones are removed from the body and flushed out along with urine, which reduces the content of water and sodium in the body. If you are following a ketogenic diet plan, always remember to take sips of water throughout the day if you want to avoid dehydration, headaches, and cramps.

Ignoring the Keto Flu

The keto flu, as we saw earlier, is a period in the initial stages of ketosis where you can experience flu-like symptoms such as headaches, nausea, fatigue, and body aches. This is mostly observed within the first two weeks of starting the keto diet. If you are unaware of the keto flu and unprepared to tackle the symptoms, you might be tricked into thinking that keto diet is complete nonsense and has caused something drastically wrong in your case. You need to know that it is just a transitional period where your body is beginning to adjust itself to the new diet regime that you have just adopted. The symptoms of keto flu can be avoided by eating foods that are rich in ions such as sodium, magnesium, and potassium.

Ignoring the Healthy Fatty Acids

Since the keto diet encourages eating a high-fat diet, you might be predisposed towards increasing your consumption of fried bacon, cheese, and cream. However, it is important to choose your fatty acids carefully before making them a staple part of your keto diet. Your diet should include an adequate amount of healthy fatty acids, such as omega-3 fatty acids, EPA, and DHA. These healthy fats are abundantly found in seafood (sardines, tuna, salmon, herring, mussels, scallops), so make sure that to include these in your diet. If you aren't a big fan of seafood, you can supplement your diet by taking cod liver oil capsules and other supplements. Healthy oils such as coconut oil, avocado oil, virgin olive oil, flaxseed oil, and chia oil are also a good source of keto-friendly fatty acids.

Not Having Enough Salt

Most people who do not follow a ketogenic diet consume more sodium than necessary in the form of processed foods and junk food. Therefore, you are probably not used to being told to eat more salt. However, if you are following a keto diet, salt is necessary. The rapid production of ketones and its subsequent removal along with urine can lower the level of sodium in the body. Another thing to remember is that on a ketogenic diet, you will be kicking out any processed or packaged foods such as chips, crackers, and cookies. This change in your diet can lower sodium, so remember to salt your food adequately to avoid health problems such as thyroid imbalance.

Not Checking with A Doctor

Many people following the keto diet are on it to manage or treat some medical conditions. You need to consult your doctor or physician before getting on the keto diet, especially if you are using medication. The dosage of some medications might need some adjustment as your body enters ketosis and shows signs of improvement. So, make sure to take a second opinion from your doctor before embarking on your keto journey.

Ignoring Your Veggies

You need to balance the intake of vegetables when you are in ketosis. Vegetables contain carbohydrates and having a few too many servings of lettuce can kick your body out of ketosis. This does not mean that you completely stop eating vegetables, as some of them are important for aiding digestion and other bodily processes. You should closely notice vegetables you are eating while following a ketogenic diet plan. Having an enough leafy greens and other veggies such as tomatoes and asparagus is necessary while you are on a ketogenic diet to make sure that your body is still getting everything that it requires to function properly.

Japanese Scrambled Eggs

Serves: 2

Ingredients:

- 2 eggs
- 6 oz. Flank steak
- 4 oz. Radishes
- 1 tsp. salt
- 1 tsp. freshly ground pepper
- 2 oz. Cheddar cheese
- 1 oz. Cubetti pancetta

Directions:

1. Place a nonstick pan over medium heat. When the pan is heated, place flank steak and pan-fry for two minutes per side. When it is cool, set aside and slice it.
2. Wash thoroughly and quarter the radishes.
3. Pan-fry the radishes and the pancetta in a cast iron skillet until the radishes turn golden brown (about 7 minutes).
4. Add sliced flank steak into the pan.
5. Break the eggs into the skillet. Add the cheese, salt, and pepper to taste.
6. Let it cook for 2 minutes.
7. Put in the oven and cook for 10 minutes; broil till the eggs are cooked to the desired doneness.
8. Serve when ready.

Ham and Cream Muffins

Serves: 7

Ingredients:

- 6 eggs
- ½ oz. Ham, diced
- 5 slices cheddar cheese, chopped
- 1 bunch medium green onions (6 green onions), minced
- 1 can tomatoes, drained, 14.5 oz.
- 1 tsp. garlic powder
- 5 tbsp. Heavy cream
- 1 tsp. kosher salt
- 1 tsp. freshly ground pepper
- 1 tsp. onion powder

Directions:

1. Add heavy cream, eggs and spices into a bowl and mix them thoroughly. Add vegetables and cheese and mix well.
2. Take your muffin pan and coat it with oil. Pour into the muffin cups.
3. Bake for 5 minutes at 350 degrees Fahrenheit.
4. Remove from the oven. Run a knife around the muffins and invert onto a plate.
5. Serve when ready.

Baked Chorizo

Serves: 4

Ingredients

- 2 tbsp. butter
- 2 garlic cloves, sliced
- 1 tsp. freshly ground black pepper
- 2 oz. cream cheese
- 1 tsp. kosher salt
- 2 oz. cremini mushrooms, chopped
- ½ cup grated cheese
- 1 onion, chopped
- ¾ cup shredded cheddar cheese
- 4 oz. pork chorizo
- ¼ cup sour cream
- 3 large eggs

Directions:

1. Take a mixture of garlic, onion and butter in a skillet and sauté in medium heat for 20 minutes.
2. Continue till the mushrooms are caramelized.
3. Stir in the chorizo. Sauté till the mushrooms are tender and the chorizo completely cooked.
4. Drain the excess grease, switch to low heat and stir in the cream cheese.
5. Whisk the eggs in a mixing bowl, add the grated and cheddar cheeses and whisk until well combined.
6. Preheat oven to 375 degrees F
7. Spread the chorizo mixture in a casserole dish, top with the egg/cheese mixture.
8. Stir well.
9. Bake uncovered for 25 minutes.
10. Garnish with the sour cream. Serve when ready.

Simple Omelet

Serves: 4

Ingredients:

- 6 eggs
- 1 tbsp. garlic powder
- 1 tbsp. kosher salt
- 1 oz. cheddar cheese
- 1 tbsp. freshly ground pepper
- 4 tsp. oil

Directions:

1. Whisk eggs in a bowl. Add heavy cream, garlic and cheese and whisk well.
2. Place a small pan over medium heat.
3. Add a tsp. of oil and let it heat.
4. Pour ¼ of the mixture into the pan.
5. Sprinkle salt and pepper. Cook until the underside is golden brown. Flip sides and cook the other side until golden brown.
6. Repeat steps 3 – 5 and make the remaining omelets.

White Creamy Avocado

Serves: 2

Ingredients:

- ¼ avocado de-seeded and de-skinned, chopped
- 4 eggs
- 3/8 cup heavy whipping cream
- 5 ice cubes
- 3/8 cup unsweetened almond milk
- Stevia or swerve to taste

Directions:

1. Add almond milk, heavy whipping cream, eggs and sweetener, heavy whipping cream, avocado and ice cubes into your blender.
2. Blend to smooth consistency.
3. Pour into glasses and serve.

Steak and Eggs

Serves: 7

Ingredients:

- ½ onion, chopped
- ½ bell pepper, chopped
- 5 eggs
- 3 oz. Cheddar cheese
- 2 lbs. lean meat, thickly sliced
- 1 pepper, sliced
- 2 tbsp. Heavy cream, whipped
- 1 tsp. garlic powder
- 1 tsp. freshly ground black pepper
- 1 tsp. kosher salt
- 1 tsp. onion powder
- 1 tsp. oil

Directions:

1. Place a pan over medium heat. Add oil. When the oil heats, add onion and bell pepper and cook until tender. Set aside.
2. Add meat into the skillet. Cook meat for 6 minutes (3 minutes per side) over high heat.
3. Meanwhile, prepare the eggs.
4. In a bowl, mix the spices, cream, and eggs.
5. Cook mixture with a non-stick pan until slightly set. Now scramble the eggs.
6. Add cheese, whisk again.
7. Serve eggs, onions, pepper and meat.

Deviled Eggs in Soy Sauce

Serves: 3

Ingredients:

- 3 large eggs, hardboiled, peeled
- ¼ cup soy sauce
- 2 ounces cream cheese, softened
- ½ cup + 2 tbsp. water
- ½ tbsp. chopped chives
- 1 clove garlic, peeled, grated
- ½ tsp. liquid stevia
- Pepper to taste
- Salt to taste
- 2 tbsp. rice vinegar

Directions:

1. Take a bowl and add vinegar, soy sauce, half a cup of water, stevia, garlic and whisk it all together.
2. Peel the eggs and place them in the marinade. Use some paper towels to cover the eggs. The towels will absorb some of the marinade but will help to keep the eggs in the marinade. Keep it in the refrigerator for a couple of hours.
3. Make sure you turn the eggs at intervals of 15-20 minutes.
4. Take the eggs out and remove them from the bowl. Pat with paper towels.
5. Cut the eggs in 2 halves, lengthwise. Scoop out the yolks and set aside the whites as well as the yolks.
6. Add cream cheese and 2 tbsp. water into a bowl. Beat thoroughly with an electric hand mixer until creamy.
7. Add yolks, salt, pepper and chives. Beat until well combined.
8. Fill the cavities of the whites with the concoction.
9. Garnish with pepper and serve in your desired style.

Classic Fried Bacon

Serves: 2

Ingredients:

- 3 thickly cut medium sliced bacon
- 1 cup chopped cabbage
- 1 tbsp. butter
- ¼ chopped carrots
- 2 tbsp. garlic powder
- 1 tbsp. freshly ground black pepper
- 1 tbsp. onion powder
- 1 tbsp. grated cheese
- 1 cup chopped cabbage
- 1 tbsp. kosher salt

Directions:

1. Take a hot cast iron pan and cook the bacon in it for 5 minutes on medium heat. Stir whenever needed. Once you are done, set it aside.
2. Turn the heat to medium high and stir the onion powder and butter for two minutes.
3. Once done, add carrots and cabbage. Cook it for 5 minutes till they become tender.
4. Turn off the heat. Proceed to stir the salt, pepper, cheese and cooked bacon.
5. Serve it hot.

Garlic Parmesan Chicken Wings

Serves: 4

Ingredients:

- 20 frozen wing sections (wings and drums)
- 1 tsp. garlic salt
- 4 tbsp. garlic infused olive oil
- 2 tsp. of garlic powder
- 1 cup Parmesan, grated

Directions:

1. Take a baking rack and place the chicken wings carefully. Use garlic salt and sprinkle it on top of the wings. Place the rack in the oven. Place a baking pan below it.
2. Bake in a preheated oven at 400°F for about 30 minutes or until done.
3. Use some garlic oil and brush over the wings.
4. Let it broil for 5 minutes until the skin turns crisp and visibly brown. Remove from the oven and place in a bowl.
5. Pour remaining garlic oil over it and toss well.
6. Sprinkle garlic powder and Parmesan and toss well.
7. Serve right away.

Egg and Quail Sandwich

Serves: 5

Ingredients:

- 5 quail eggs
- 5 slices bacon
- 2 slices cheddar cheese
- Salt to taste
- Pepper to taste

Almond buns:

- 6 tbsp. almond flour
- 1 large egg
- 2 ½ tbsp. unsalted butter
- ¾ tsp. baking powder
- ¾ tsp. Splenda

Directions:

1. Mix all the ingredients for almond buns in a bowl.
2. Divide the almond bun mixture into 5 portions and place in a whoopee pie pan.
3. Bake for 10 minutes at 350 degrees F
4. Cook the quail eggs to the desired doneness and season with salt and pepper. Cook the sliced bacon.
5. Take each almond bun and top it with half a slice of bacon, one quail egg, and 1/4th cheese slice.
6. Serve it when ready.

Green Beans with Cream

Serves: 4

Ingredients:

- 1 lb. fresh green beans, trimmed and rinsed
- 1/2 tsp. grated lemon zest
- 1/4 tsp. pepper
- 1/2 tsp. sea salt
- 1 cup heavy cream
- 3 oz. butter

Directions:

1. Take a pan and melt some butter over it. Set the heat at medium.
2. Add green beans into the pan and sauté for 4-5 minutes. Add pepper and salt to taste.
3. Add heavy cream into the pan and lower the heat to medium-low heat. Let it simmer for 2 minutes.
4. Garnish with lemon zest and serve for a delicious experience.

Chicken Fajitas

Serves: 6

Ingredients:

- 1 ½ lbs. chicken tenders
- 1 tsp. chicken seasoning
- 1 tbsp. olive oil
- 2 tbsp. BBQ sauce, unsweetened

Directions:

1. Add all ingredients except oil in a zip-lock bag.
2. Seal bag. Shake well and place in the fridge for 2-3 hours.
3. Heat oil in a pan over medium heat.
4. Cook chicken tenders in a pan until completely cooked.
5. Serve and enjoy.

Mashed Cauliflower Magic

Serves: 4

Ingredients:

- 1 lb. cauliflower, cut into florets
- 1 tbsp. lemon juice
- ¼ tsp. onion powder
- 3 oz. Parmesan cheese, grated
- ½ tsp. garlic powder
- Pepper according to taste
- Salt according to taste
- 4 oz. butter

Directions:

1. Boil cauliflower florets until tender. Drain well.
2. Add cooked cauliflower into the blender with remaining ingredients and blend until smooth.
3. Serve and enjoy with your loved ones.

Parmesan Chicken

Serves: 2

Ingredients:

- 0.5 lb. chicken breasts, skinless and boneless
- 1/2 tsp. garlic powder
- 1/4 cup Parmesan cheese, grated
- 1/4 tsp. onion powder
- 1/4 cup mayonnaise
- 1/2 tsp. poultry seasoning
- 1/4 tsp. pepper

Directions:

1. Preheat the oven to 375 F.
2. In a small bowl, mix mayonnaise, garlic powder, onion powder, poultry seasoning, and pepper.
3. Place chicken in greased baking dish.
4. Spread mayonnaise mixture over chicken then sprinkle cheese.
5. Bake for 35 minutes.
6. Serve and enjoy.

Broccoli Roast

Serves: 4

Ingredients:

- 2 lbs. broccoli, cut into florets
- 3 tbsp. olive oil
- 1 tbsp. lemon juice
- 1/4 cup Parmesan cheese, grated
- 3 garlic cloves, sliced
- ½ tsp. red pepper flakes
- 1/4 tsp. pepper
- 1/4 tsp. salt

Directions:

1. Preheat the oven to 425 F.
2. Add broccoli, pepper, salt, garlic, and oil in large bowl and toss well.
3. Spread broccoli on baking tray and roast in for 20 minutes.
4. Add lemon juice, grated cheese, red pepper flakes and almonds over broccoli and toss well.
5. Serve and enjoy with your friends and family.

Curried Coconut Chicken

Serves: 8

Ingredients:

- 6 chicken thighs
- 14.5 oz. coconut milk
- ½ tbsp. curry powder
- 3 garlic cloves, minced
- 1 onion, sliced
- 1 tbsp. olive oil
- 2 green onions, sliced
- 3 tbsp. chopped fresh cilantro
- 3 cups chicken broth
- 1/4 tsp. pepper
- 1 tsp. salt

Directions:

1. Place a skillet over medium heat. Add oil. Add onion. Sauté until translucent. Add garlic and stir for a few seconds until aromatic. Season chicken with salt and pepper and place in the skillet. Cook until brown all over. Add
2. Add curry powder and broth and cook until chicken is tender.
3. Add coconut milk and simmer for a few minutes.
4. Serve and enjoy.

Roasted Pepper Chicken

Serves: 4

Ingredients:

- 4 chicken breasts, skinless and boneless
- 1 1/2 tsp. Italian seasoning
- 2/3 cup red peppers, roasted and chopped
- 3/4 cup heavy cream
- 3 garlic cloves, minced
- 4 tbsp. olive oil
- 1/2 tsp. salt

Directions:

1. Add roasted red pepper, garlic, oil, 1 tsp. Italian seasoning, pepper, and salt into the blender and blend until smooth.
2. Season chicken with remaining seasoning and cook in a pan over medium heat for 7-8 minutes on each side.
3. Transfer chicken to a plate.
4. Pour red pepper mixture into the pan and cook for 2 minutes.
5. Add heavy cream and stir well.
6. Return chicken to the pan stir well to coat with sauce.
7. Serve and enjoy.

Pan Fried Pork Chops

Serves: 2

Ingredients:

- 2 pork chops, boneless
- 1/3 tsp. garlic powder
- 1 tbsp. olive oil
- 1/3 tsp. pepper
- 1/3tsp. onion powder
- Salt

Directions:

1. Take an iron skillet and heat oil in it on high heat
2. Season pork chops with garlic powder, onion powder, pepper, and salt and place in the skillet.
3. Sear pork chops for about 3-4 minutes on each side.
4. Serve and enjoy.

Pesto Flavored Chicken with Asparagus

Serves: 3

Ingredients:

- 1 lb. chicken thighs, skinless, boneless, and cut into pieces
- 3/4 lb. asparagus, trimmed and cut in half
- 2 tbsp. olive oil
- 1 3/4 cups grape tomatoes, halved
- 1/4 cup basil pesto
- Pepper
- Salt

Directions:

1. Heat oil in a pan over medium heat.
2. Add chicken to the pan and season with pepper and salt and cook for 5-8 minutes.
3. Add pesto and asparagus and cook for 2-3 minutes.
4. Remove pan from heat and add tomatoes and stir well.
5. Serve and enjoy.

Juicy & Tender Baked Pork Chops

Serves: 4

Ingredients:

- 4 pork chops, boneless
- 2 tbsp. olive oil
- ½ tsp. Italian seasoning
- ½ tsp. paprika
- ½ tsp. garlic powder
- ¼ tsp. pepper
- ½ tsp. sea salt

Directions:

1. Preheat the oven to 375 F.
2. In a small bowl, mix garlic powder, paprika, Italian seasoning, pepper, and salt.
3. Brush pork chops with oil and rub with garlic powder mixture.
4. Place pork chops onto a baking tray and bake in preheated oven for 30-35 minutes.
5. Serve and enjoy.

Simple Grilled Pork Tenderloin

Serves: 16

Ingredients:

- 4 lbs. pork tenderloin
- 4 tbsp. olive oil
- 4 tbsp. ranch dressing mix
- Salt according to taste

Directions:

1. Preheat the grill to 350 F.
2. Brush pork belly with oil and use ranch dressing for seasoning.
3. Place pork on the grill. Cook it for 30 minutes. Turn tenderloin every 10 minutes.
4. Slice and serve to your family.

Pork Chops with Garlic and Rosemary

Serves: 4

Ingredients:

- 2 garlic cloves, minced
- 1 tsp. dried rosemary, crushed
- 4 pork chops, boneless
- ¼ tsp. onion powder
- ¼ tsp. pepper
- ¼ tsp. sea salt

Directions:

1. Preheat the oven to 425 F.
2. Season pork chops with onion powder, pepper and salt.
3. Mix rosemary and garlic together and rub all over pork chops.
4. Place the pork chops on a baking tray and roast for 10 minutes.
5. Set temperature 350 F and roast for 25 minutes more.
6. Serve and enjoy with your family.

Yummy Minced Pork Magic

Serves: 3

Ingredients:

- 14 oz. minced pork
- 1/4 cup green bell pepper, chopped
- 1/2 onion, chopped
- 2 tbsp. water
- ¼ tsp. cumin powder
- 3/4 cup ketchup, sugar-free
- 1/2 tbsp. olive oil
- Pepper
- Salt

Directions:

1. Heat oil in pan over medium heat.
2. Add pepper and onion and sauté until soften.
3. Add meat, pepper, cumin powder, and salt and cook until browned.
4. Add water and ketchup and stir well. Bring to boil.
5. Serve and enjoy.

Baked Scrumptious Wings

Serves: 8

Ingredients:

- 4 lbs. chicken wings
- 2 tbsp. lemon pepper seasoning
- 4 tbsp. butter, melted
- 8 tbsp. olive oil

Directions:

1. Preheat the oven to 400 F.
2. Toss chicken wings with olive oil.
3. Arrange chicken wings on a baking tray and bake for 50 minutes.
4. In a small bowl, mix lemon pepper seasoning and butter.
5. Remove wings from oven and brush with butter and seasoning mixture.
6. Serve and enjoy with everyone.

Creamy Cabbage

Serves: 8

Ingredients:

- 1 cabbage head, shredded
- 2 onions, sliced
- 6 garlic cloves, chopped
- 2 bell peppers, cut into strips
- 1/2 tsp. garlic powder
- 4 tbsp. butter
- 1/2 tsp. onion powder
- 1 tsp. pepper
- 2 tsp. kosher salt
- 6 oz. cream cheese

Directions:

1. Take a pan and melt some butter over it. Set the heat at medium.
2. Add garlic and onion and sauté for 5 minutes.
3. Add cabbage and bell pepper and cook for 5 minutes.
4. Add remaining ingredients and stir well.
5. Serve and enjoy with your friends and family.

Spinach Broccoli and Chicken

Serves: 4

Ingredients:

- 1 lb. chicken breasts, cut into pieces
- 4 oz. cream cheese
- 1/2 cup Parmesan cheese, shredded
- 2 cups baby spinach
- 2 cup broccoli florets
- 1 tomato, chopped
- 2 garlic cloves, minced
- 1 tsp. Italian seasoning
- 2 tbsp. olive oil
- Pepper
- Salt

Directions:

1. Take some oil and heat it in a saucepan over medium to high heat.
2. In the next step, add some chicken, season with pepper, Italian seasoning, and salt and sauté until chicken cooked through, for roughly 5 minutes.
3. Add garlic and sauté for a minute.
4. Add cream cheese, Parmesan cheese, spinach, broccoli, and tomato and cook for 3-4 minutes more.
5. Serve and enjoy with your friends and family.

Delicious Pumpkin Risotto

Serves: 2

Ingredients:

- 1/2 cup pumpkin, grated
- 2 tbsp. butter
- 1 cup water
- 2 cups cauliflower, grated
- 4 garlic cloves, chopped
- 1/4 tsp. cinnamon
- Pepper according to taste
- Salt according to taste

Directions:

1. Take a pan and melt some butter over it on medium to high heat.
2. Add garlic, cauliflower, cinnamon and pumpkin into the pan and season with pepper and salt.
3. Cook until lightly softened. Take some water and add it to the mixture. Keep cooking until it is done.
4. Serve and enjoy with your family and friends.

Delicious Bacon and Chicken Delight

Serves: 6

Ingredients:

- 2 1/2 lbs. chicken breasts, cut in half
- 1/2 tsp. paprika
- 1/2 tsp. onion powder
- 4 oz. cheddar cheese, shredded
- 1/2 tsp. garlic powder
- 1/2 lb. bacon, cut into strips
- Pepper according to taste
- Salt according to taste

Directions:

1. Preheat the oven to 400 F.
2. In a small bowl, mix paprika, onion powder, garlic powder, pepper, and salt.
3. Rub chicken with spice mixture.
4. Place chicken on a baking tray and top each with bacon piece.
5. Bake for 30 minutes. Remove from oven and sprinkle with cheese and bake for 10 minutes.
6. Serve and enjoy.

Noodles with Rutabaga

Serves: 8

Ingredients:

- 50 oz. rutabaga, peel, cut and make into spirals using slicer
- 1 tbsp. chili powder
- 2/3 cup olive oil
- 1 tsp. garlic powder
- 1/2 tsp. onion powder
- 1 tsp. salt

Directions:

1. Preheat the oven to 450 F.
2. Add all ingredients into the large bowl and toss well.
3. Spread rutabaga mixture on a baking tray and bake for 10 minutes.
4. Serve and enjoy a healthy meal with your guests.

Chicken with Mexican Touch

Serves: 6

Ingredients:

- 1 1/2 cup cheddar cheese
- 2 cups chicken, cooked and shredded
- 3/4 cup chicken broth
- 14 oz. Rotel tomatoes
- 2 garlic cloves, minced
- 1/2 cup Monterey jack cheese
- 1/3 cup green pepper, diced
- 1 onion, diced
- 2 tsp. taco seasoning
- 12 oz. cauliflower rice
- 1 tbsp. butter

Directions:

1. Melt butter in a pan over medium heat.
2. Add garlic, pepper, and onion and sauté until softened.
3. Steam cauliflower rice according to packet instructions.
4. Add seasoning, broth, cauliflower rice, and Rotel tomatoes to the pan.
5. Stir well and cook for 10 minutes.
6. Add chicken and cook for 5 minutes.
7. Top with cheese and cook until cheese is melted.
8. Serve and enjoy.

Chicken and Cheese Casserole

Serves: 8

Ingredients:

- 2 lbs. chicken, cooked and shredded
- 5 oz. ham, cut into small pieces
- 5 oz. Swiss cheese
- 3/4 tbsp. Dijon mustard
- 5 oz. cream cheese, softened
- 4 oz. butter, melted
- 1 oz. fresh lemon juice
- ½ tsp. salt

Directions:

1. Preheat the oven to 350 F.
2. Add chicken in a baking dish then carefully place ham pieces on top of it.
3. Add butter, lemon juice, mustard, cream cheese, and salt into the blender and blend until smooth.
4. Pour butter mixture over chicken and ham mixture.
5. Arrange cheese slices on top and bake for 40 minutes.
6. Serve and enjoy a delicious meal with your loved ones.

Cheesy Loaded Jalapenos

Serves: 24

Ingredients:

- 12 jalapenos, halved
- 6 tbsp. green onion, sliced
- 1/2 cup cheddar cheese, shredded
- 1 tsp. dried basil
- 1/2 tsp. garlic powder
- 6 oz. cream cheese
- 1 tsp. dried oregano
- 1/2 tsp. salt
- 1 cup chicken, cooked and shredded

Directions:

1. Preheat the oven to 390 F.
2. Mix all ingredients in a bowl except jalapenos.
3. Stuff chicken mixture into each jalapeno halved and place on a baking tray.
4. Bake for 25 minutes.
5. Serve and bask in the deliciousness with your loved ones!

Asian Garlic Chicken

Serves: 12

Ingredients:

- 3 lbs. chicken breasts, skinless and boneless
- 4 tbsp. water
- 4 tbsp. soy sauce
- 1 onion, chopped
- 3 tsp. red pepper flakes
- 4 garlic cloves, minced
- 1 tsp. ground ginger

Directions:

1. Place chicken into the crockpot.
2. Add remaining ingredients on top of chicken.
3. Cover and cook on high for 4 hours.
4. Shred the chicken using a fork.
5. Serve and relish the taste with your loved ones!

Cheese and Olive Omelet Style Eggs

Serves: 6

Ingredients:

- 6 large eggs
- 3 oz. cheese
- 16 olives, pitted
- 3 tbsp. butter
- 3 tbsp. olive oil
- 1 1/2 tsp. herb
- 1 tsp. salt

Directions:

1. Add all ingredients except butter in a bowl whisk well until frothy.
2. Melt butter in a pan over medium heat.
3. Pour egg mixture onto hot pan and spread evenly.
4. Cover and cook for 3 minutes.
5. Turn omelet to other side and cook for 2 minutes more.
6. Serve and enjoy this flavorful brunch style dish!

Creamy Chicken Mushrooms

Serves: 8

Ingredients:

- 4 lbs. chicken breasts, halved
- 1/2 cup sun-dried tomatoes
- 14 oz. mushrooms, sliced
- 1 cup mayonnaise
- 2 tsp. salt

Directions:

1. Preheat the oven to 400 F.
2. Place chicken breasts into the greased baking dish and top with sun-dried tomatoes, mushrooms, mayonnaise, and salt. Mix well.
3. Bake in the oven for 30 minutes.
4. Serve and enjoy with your loved ones!

Mashed Broccoli and Cauliflower Delight

Serves: 8

Ingredients:

- 4 cups cauliflower florets
- 4 cups broccoli florets
- 4 garlic cloves, peeled
- 1/2 tsp. onion powder
- 2 tbsp. olive oil
- 2 tsp. pepper
- 1 tsp. salt

Directions:

1. Take some olive oil and let it heat on medium temperature on a pan.
2. Add cauliflower, broccoli, and salt in a pan and sauté until softened.
3. Transfer vegetables and garlic to the food processor and process until smooth.
4. Season with onion powder, pepper and salt.
5. Serve and enjoy.

Cheesy Bacon Chicken

Serves: 4

Ingredients:

- 3 chicken breasts, skinless and boneless
- 1/2 cup chicken broth
- 1/2 tsp. garlic, minced
- 1/8 tsp. thyme
- 1/4 tsp. Rosemary
- 1/4 tsp. poultry seasoning
- 1/4 cup cheddar cheese
- 1 oz. cream cheese
- 1/3 cup heavy cream
- 2 bacon pieces, cooked and crumbled
- 1 1/2 tbsp. butter
- Pepper according to taste
- Salt according to taste

Directions:

1. Place a large skillet over medium heat. Add butter. When butter melts, add chicken and cook until brown all over.
2. Add chicken broth, garlic, thyme, rosemary and poultry seasoning and mix well.
3. Cover and cook until chicken is cooked through.
4. Add cream cheese and cream and stir well to combine.
5. Remove chicken with a slotted spoon and place on a plate. Shred the chicken using a pair of forks.
6. Transfer chicken mixture into the greased casserole dish.
7. Top with cheddar cheese and broil for 4 minutes. Sprinkle bacon on top.
8. Serve and enjoy with your loved ones!

Flavored Zucchini

Serves: 9

Ingredients:

- 4 cups zucchini, sliced
- 1 1/2 cups shredded pepper jack cheese
- 2 tbsp. butter
- 1 onion, sliced
- ¼ tsp. onion powder
- 1/2 tsp. garlic powder
- 1/2 cup heavy cream
- Pepper according to taste
- Salt according to taste

Directions:

1. Preheat the oven to 375 F.
2. Place sliced onion and zucchini in a baking pan and season with pepper and salt.
3. Sprinkle 1/2-cup cheese on top of onion and zucchini.
4. In a microwave safe dish, combine heavy cream, butter, garlic powder, and onion powder and microwave for 1 minute.
5. Pour heavy cream mixture over sliced zucchini and onion.
6. Bake for 45 minutes.
7. Serve and enjoy with your loved ones.

Delicious Chicken Strips

Serves: 4

Ingredients:

- 1 ½ lbs. chicken tenders
- 1 tsp. chicken seasoning
- 1 tbsp. olive oil
- 2 tbsp. BBQ sauce, unsweetened

Directions:

1. Add all ingredients except oil in a zip-lock bag.
2. Seal bag and shake well and place in the fridge for 2-3 hours.
3. Heat oil in a pan over medium heat.
4. Add chicken and cook until completely cooked.
5. Serve and enjoy with your love's ones!

Stir Fried Mushroom and Broccoli Magic

Serves: 4

Ingredients:

- 2 cups broccoli, cut into florets
- 1 1/2 tsp. fresh ginger, grated
- 1/4 tsp. red pepper flakes
- 2 cups mushrooms, sliced
- 2 garlic cloves, minced
- 1 small onion, chopped
- 2 tbsp. balsamic vinegar
- 1/2 tbsp. sesame seeds
- 2 tbsp. soy sauce, low sodium
- 1/4 cup cashews
- 1 medium carrot, shredded
- 3 tbsp. water

Directions:

1. Take a large pan and heat over high heat.
2. Add broccoli, water, red pepper, mushrooms, ginger, garlic, and onion into the pan and cook until the mixture has softened.
3. Add carrots, soy sauce, vinegar, and cashews. Stir well and simmer for 2 minutes.
4. Garnish with sesame seeds.
5. Serve and enjoy with your loved ones!

Vegetable Quiche

Serves: 6

Ingredients:

- 8 eggs
- 1 onion, chopped
- 1 cup Parmesan cheese, grated
- 1 cup unsweetened coconut milk
- 1 cup tomatoes, chopped
- 1 cup zucchini, chopped
- 1 tbsp. butter
- 1/2 tsp. pepper
- 1 tsp. salt

Directions:

1. Preheat the oven to 400 F.
2. Melt butter in an ovenproof pan over medium heat then add onion and sauté until onion soften.
3. Add tomatoes and zucchini to pan and sauté for 4 minutes. Remove from heat.
4. Beat eggs with cheese, milk, pepper and salt in a bowl.
5. Pour egg mixture over vegetables and bake in oven for 30 minutes.
6. Slice properly and serve.

Pumpkin Muffins

Serves: 10

Ingredients:

- 4 eggs
- 1/2 cup pumpkin puree
- 1 tsp. pumpkin pie spice
- 1/2 cup almond flour
- 1 tbsp. baking powder
- 1 tsp. vanilla
- 1/3 cup coconut oil, melted
- 2/3 cup swerve
- 1/2 cup coconut flour
- 1/2 tsp. sea salt

Directions:

1. Preheat the oven to 350 F.
2. In a large bowl, stir together coconut flour, pumpkin pie spice, baking powder, swerve, almond flour, and sea salt.
3. Stir in eggs, vanilla, coconut oil, and pumpkin puree until well combined.
4. Pour batter into the greased muffin tray and bake in oven for 25 minutes.
5. Serve and enjoy.

Roasted Green Beans

Serves: 4

Ingredients:

- 1 lb. frozen green beans
- ¼ tsp. red pepper flakes
- 1/4 tsp. garlic powder
- 2 tbsp. olive oil
- 1/2 tsp. onion powder
- 1/2 tsp. pepper
- 1/2 tsp. salt

Directions:

1. Preheat the oven to 425 F.
2. In a large bowl, add all ingredients and mix well.
3. Spread the mixture on a baking tray and bake for 30 minutes.
4. Serve and enjoy.

Broccoli Fries

Serves: 4

Ingredients:

- 2 egg whites
- 2 cups broccoli florets, steamed
- 1/4 cup almond flour
- 1 cup cheddar cheese, shredded
- 1/8 tsp. salt

Directions:

1. Preheat the oven to 350 F.
2. Add broccoli in bowl and mash using masher.
3. Add remaining ingredients to the broccoli and mix well.
4. Drop about 20 scoops onto baking tray and press lightly down.
5. Bake in preheated oven for 20 minutes.
6. Serve and enjoy.

Quiche with Cheese and Spinach

Serves: 6

Ingredients:

- 8 eggs
- 2 cups fresh spinach
- 1/2 cup feta cheese, crumbled
- 1/2 cup Parmesan cheese, shredded
- 1/4 cup cheddar cheese, shredded
- 3 garlic cloves, minced
- 2 cups unsweetened almond milk
- 1/4 tsp. salt

Directions:

1. Preheat the oven to 350 F.
2. In a large bowl, whisk together eggs and almond milk.
3. Add spinach, Parmesan cheese, feta cheese, garlic, and salt and stir well to combine.
4. Spray an ovenproof skillet with cooking spray. Place the skillet over medium heat. When the pan is heated, pour egg mixture into the pan.
5. Sprinkle shredded cheddar cheese over the top of egg mixture. When the egg is slightly set around the edges, turn off the heat.
6. Transfer into the oven and bake for 15 minutes or until set.
7. Serve and enjoy with your family and friends.

Cheese Almond Pancakes

Serves: 4

Ingredients:

- 4 eggs
- 1/4 tsp. cinnamon
- 1/2 cup cream cheese
- 1/2 cup almond flour
- 1 tbsp. butter

Directions:

1. Add eggs, cinnamon, cream cheese and almond flour into the blender and blend until combined.
2. Place a pan over medium heat.
3. Add ¼ tsp. of butter into the pan. When butter melts,
4. Pour ¼ of the batter and cook for 2 minutes on each side. Remove onto a plate.
5. Repeat steps 3 – 4 and make the remaining pancakes.
6. Serve and enjoy with your friends and family.

Cauliflower Frittata

Serves: 2

Ingredients:

- 2 eggs
- 1 tbsp. onion, diced
- ½ cup cauliflower rice
- 2 tbsp. olive oil
- ½ tsp. turmeric
- Pepper according to taste
- Salt according to taste

Directions:

1. Add all ingredients except oil into the bowl and mix well to combine.
2. Warm oil in a pan and set the temperature to medium.
3. Pour the mixture into the hot oil pan and cook for 3-4 minutes or until lightly golden brown.
4. Serve and enjoy with your family and friends.

Chia Spinach Pancakes

Serves: 6

Ingredients:

- 4 eggs
- ½ cup coconut flour
- 1 cup coconut milk
- ¼ cup chia seeds
- 1 cup spinach, chopped
- 1 tsp. baking soda
- ½ tsp. pepper
- ½ tsp. salt
- Butter, to fry

Directions:

1. Whisk eggs in a bowl until frothy.
2. Combine all dry ingredients and add in egg mixture and whisk until smooth. Add spinach and stir well.
3. Grease pan with a little butter and heat over medium heat.
4. Pour 3-4 tbsp. of batter onto the pan and make pancake.
5. Cook pancake until lightly golden brown from both the sides. Remove the pancake and place on a plate.
6. Repeat steps 3 – 5 and make the remaining pancakes.
7. Serve and enjoy.

Feta Kale Frittata

Serves: 8

Ingredients:

- 8 eggs, beaten
- 4 oz. feta cheese, crumbled
- 6 oz. bell pepper, roasted and diced
- 5 oz. baby kale
- 1/4 cup green onion, sliced
- 2 tsp. olive oil

Directions:

1. Take a pan and warm some oil in it on medium heat.
2. Add kale to the pan and sauté for 4-5 minutes or until softened.
3. Spray slow cooker with cooking spray.
4. Add cooked kale into the slow cooker.
5. Add green onion and bell pepper into the slow cooker.
6. Pour beaten eggs into the slow cooker and stir well to combine.
7. Sprinkle crumbled feta cheese.
8. Cook on low for 2 hours or until frittata is set.
9. Serve and enjoy.

Salted Protein Muffins

Serves: 12

Ingredients:

- 8 eggs
- 2 scoop vanilla protein powder
- 8 oz. cream cheese
- 4 tbsp. butter, melted

Directions:

1. In a large bowl, combine cream cheese and melted butter.
2. Add eggs and protein powder and whisk until well combined.
3. Pour batter into a 12 counts greased muffin pan.
4. Bake at 350 F for 25 minutes.
5. Serve and enjoy with your friends and family.

Healthy Waffles

Serves: 4

Ingredients:

- 8 drops liquid stevia
- 1/2 tsp. baking soda
- 1 tbsp. chia seeds
- 1/4 cup water
- 2 tbsp. sunflower seed butter
- 1 tsp. cinnamon
- 1 avocado, peel, pitted and mashed
- 1 tsp. vanilla
- 1 tbsp. lemon juice
- 3 tbsp. coconut flour

Directions:

1. Preheat the waffle iron.
2. In a small bowl, add water and chia seeds and soak for 5 minutes.
3. Mash together sunflower seed butter, lemon juice, vanilla, stevia, chia mixture, and avocado.
4. Mix cinnamon, baking soda, and coconut flour.
5. Add wet ingredients to the dry ingredients and mix well.
6. Pour ¼ of the waffle mixture into the hot waffle iron and cook on each side for 3-5 minutes.
7. Repeat step 6 and make the remaining waffles.
8. Serve and enjoy.

Cheese Zucchini Eggplant

Serves: 8

Ingredients:

- 1 eggplant, peeled and cut in 1-inch cubes
- 1 ½ cup spaghetti sauce
- 1 onion, sliced
- 1 medium zucchini, cut into 1-inch pieces
- 1/2 cup Parmesan cheese, shredded

Directions:

1. Preheat the oven to 375 F
2. Add all ingredients into a baking dish and stir well.
3. Cover the dish with foil.
4. Bake for 20 minutes. Uncover and bake until cooked through.
5. Stir thoroughly and serve when ready!

Coconut Kale Muffins

Serves: 8

Ingredients:

- 6 eggs
- 1/2 cup unsweetened coconut milk
- 1 cup kale, chopped
- ¼ tsp. garlic powder
- ¼ tsp. paprika
- 1/4 cup green onion, chopped
- Pepper according to taste
- Salt according to taste

Directions:

1. Preheat the oven to 350 F.
2. Add all ingredients into the bowl and whisk well.
3. Pour mixture into the greased muffin tray and bake in oven for 30 minutes.
4. Serve and enjoy.

Buffalo Chicken

Serves: 4

Ingredients:

- 1 Tbsp. butter, chopped
- 6 frozen chicken breasts
- 1 bottle of cayenne peppers sauce
- 1 cup of your favorite garlic sauce

Directions:

1. Preheat oven to 375 F
2. Place chicken in a greased baking dish. Pour the hot sauce over chicken and sprinkle ranch over top.
3. Scatter button on top.
4. Bake for 30 minutes or until chicken is cooked through.

Zucchini Soup with Crunchy Cured Ham

Serves: 4

Ingredients:

- 2 leeks (white part only)
- 12 ounces zucchinis
- 10 ounces summer squash
- 3 tbsp. virgin olive oil
- 5 cups water
- Salt to taste
- 2 slices cured ham
- Black pepper according to taste

Directions:

1. Cut the leeks into thin slices and chop the zucchinis and summer squash into cubes.
2. In a large saucepan, heat the olive oil and add the leeks. Cook the leeks until they are soft, stirring gently.
3. Add in the chopped zucchinis and summer squash and cook them for about 5 minutes.
4. Add in water and bring to the boil for about 15 minutes.
5. Blend or process the soup in batches until smooth.
6. Season the soup to taste.
7. In a frying pan cook ham until crispy.
8. Divide the soup amongst the serving bowls and sprinkle with the crunchy ham strips and some black pepper.
9. Serve hot.

Non-Vegetarian Endive Bowl

Serves: 6

Ingredients

- 1 endive head, cut into wide strips
- 1 1/2 lbs. skinless boneless chicken thighs 1
- 1 Tbsp. dried oregano
- 2 cups chopped onions
- 4 celery stalks, chopped
- 4 garlic cloves, chopped
- 1 cup diced tomatoes in juice
- 2 Tbsp. olive oil
- 8 cups water

Directions:

1. Take a big saucepan. Warm oil after setting stove to medium to high heat.
2. Sprinkle the chicken with salt, pepper, and oregano. Add chicken into a saucepan.
3. Mix in onions, celery and garlic. Sauté until vegetables begin to soften, about four to five minutes.
4. Stir in tomatoes. Add broth; bring to boil. Turn down the heat to a medium flame; let it simmer until vegetables and chicken are tender, about 15 minutes.
5. Add endives; simmer until wilted, about 3 minutes. Use salt and pepper to season the dish.
6. Use a ladle to serve into bowls and serve hot.

Creamy Tuscan Garlic Chicken

Serves: 8

Ingredients:

- 3 pounds boneless, skinless, chicken breasts, thinly sliced
- 2 cups heavy cream
- 2 tsp. garlic powder
- 1 cup Parmesan cheese
- 1 cup sun-dried tomatoes
- 4 tbsp. olive oil
- 1 cup chicken broth
- 2 tsp. Italian seasoning
- 2 cups chopped spinach

Directions:

1. Place a large skillet over medium heat. Add half the oil. When the oil is heated, add half the chicken and cook until brown all over. Remove chicken and set aside on a plate.
2. Repeat the previous step and cook the remaining chicken.
3. Add cream, garlic powder, broth, Parmesan cheese and Italian seasoning into the pan. Whisk well. When the mixture begins to simmer, stir in the spinach and sun-dried tomatoes and cook until spinach wilts.
4. Place the cooked chicken in the skillet and stir until well coated. You can serve it over zucchini noodles.

Shrimp with Cauliflower "Grits" and Arugula

Serves: 8

Ingredients:

For spicy shrimp:

- 2 pounds peeled, deveined shrimp
- 4 tsp. garlic powder
- 2 tbsp. extra-virgin olive oil
- 2 tbsp. paprika
- 1 tsp. cayenne pepper
- Salt to taste
- Freshly ground pepper to taste

For cauliflower grits:

- 2 tbsp. unsalted butter
- 2 cups whole milk
- Salt to taste
- Freshly ground pepper to taste
- 8 cups riced cauliflower
- 1 cup crumbled goat cheese

For garlic arugula:

- 2 tbsp. extra-virgin olive oil
- 8 cups baby arugula
- 6 cloves garlic, thinly sliced
- Salt to taste
- Freshly ground pepper to taste

Directions:

1. For spicy shrimp: Take a large Ziploc bag and place the shrimp in it. Add paprika, cayenne and garlic powder into a bowl and stir. Sprinkle over the shrimp. Seal the bag and turn the bag around a few times until the shrimp are well coated. Chill for 15 minutes.
2. To make cauliflower grits: Place a large pot over medium heat. Add butter. When butter melts, add cauliflower and stir-fry for a couple of minutes.

3. Add half the milk and cook until slightly dry. Add rest of the milk and simmer until creamy.
4. Add goat cheeses, salt and pepper and mix well. Turn off the heat. Cover and set aside.
5. For garlic arugula: Place another skillet over medium heat. Add half the oil. When the oil is heated, add garlic and cook for a few seconds until aromatic.
6. Stir in the arugula and cook until it wilts. Add salt and pepper to taste. Transfer into a bowl.
7. Add remaining oil. When the oil is heated, add shrimp and cook until pink. Add salt and pepper to taste.
8. To assemble: Place equal amount of grits in 8 plates. Divide the arugula and place over the grits. Divide the shrimp and place over the arugula.
9. Serve right away.

Garlic Butter Brazilian Steak

Serves: 8

Ingredients:

- 12 medium cloves garlic, peeled, smashed
- 3-pound skirt steak, trimmed, cut into 8 pieces
- 4 tbsp. canola oil or vegetable oil
- 2 tbsp. chopped fresh flat-leaf parsley
- Kosher salt to taste
- Freshly ground pepper to taste
- ½ cup unsalted butter

Directions:

1. Place garlic on your cutting board. Sprinkle a little salt over it. Mince the garlic with a sharp knife.
2. Dry the steak by patting with paper towels. Sprinkle salt and pepper liberally over the steak.
3. Place a large heavy bottomed skillet over medium-high heat. Add oil. When the oil is heated, place the steak in the pan and cook until the underside is brown. Flip sides and cook the other side until brown. Turn off the heat.
4. Remove steak with a slotted spoon and place on your cutting board.
5. To make garlic butter: Place another skillet over medium heat. Add butter. When butter melts, add garlic and sauté until light golden brown. Add salt to taste. Turn off the heat.
6. When the steak is cool enough to handle, cut into slices.
7. Divide into plates. Drizzle garlic butter on the steak. Garnish with parsley and serve.

Delicious Seafood Dip

Serves: 8

Ingredients:

- 1/3 lb. shrimp, make sure it is cooked
- 1 tbsp. butter
- 1 cup of jack pepper cheese
- 2 oz. cream cheese
- 1 garlic minced clove
- 1/4 cup minced spinach
- 1/4 cup minced onion
- 2 oz. crab meat
- 2 oz. can of green chilies
- 1/3 tsp. old bay seasoning

Directions:

1. Preheat the oven to 425 F.
2. Take a pan and heat it on medium heat and melt some butter in it.
3. Once the butter is melted add some garlic, spinach, old bay seasoning, crab meat, shrimp and chilies and cook for 4-5 minutes in the pan.
4. Add half-cup pepper jack cheese and cream cheese and add it to the mixture.
5. Use the leftover cheese as topping. Let it cook for 5 minutes.
6. Serve and enjoy the delicious evening snack with your loved ones.

Garlic Cookies with Cheddar

Serves: 9

Ingredients:

- 1/4 tsp. xanthan gum
- ½ tsp. sea salt
- 1 1/2 ounces keto friendly cheese, shredded
- 1 cup almond flour, divided
- 1 ½ tbsp. butter
- 1 large egg, whisked
- 2-ounce cream cheese
- 1/2 tsp. granulated garlic
- ½ tsp. baking soda

Directions:

1. For this dish you will need a food processor. Take ½ cup almond flour and cheese and add to the processor. Let it pulse until it develops a fine texture.
2. Take a microwave safe mixing bowl and mix cream cheese and butter together. Put it into the microwave. Let it microwave on high for about 30 seconds.
3. Take out from the microwave and beat the mixture until it becomes smooth.
4. Add baking soda, garlic, salt and xanthan gum to the egg and whisk well. Use some flour mixture and add to the mixture. Start folding. Use the leftover flour to add to the dough.
5. Use a parchment paper to line the baking sheet. Take a tbsp. full of dough and place on the baking dish and use pressure to flatten it to the shape of a biscuit. Repeat this process with a gap of about an inch between biscuits.
6. Bake in a preheated oven at 325° F for 20 to 25 minutes until light golden brown on top. Remove the mixture from oven and let it simmer down for a while.
7. Serve immediately while it is warm and delicious.
8. Transfer leftovers once they are entirely cooled into an airtight container. Store at room temperature.
9. It can be preserved for 4-5 days.

Yogurt Dip

Serves: 4

Ingredients:

- 1 tbsp. olive oil
- ½ tbsp. apple cider vinegar
- 1 tsp. minced fresh thyme leaves
- Freshly ground pepper to taste
- 1 onion, thinly sliced
- 1 cup Greek yogurt
- Keto friendly crackers
- Vegetable sticks like cucumber, celery etc., to serve
- Salt according to taste.

Directions:

1. Take a pan and heat it on medium flame. Once heated, put oil in the pan. When the oil is heated, add onion, thyme, salt, and pepper and stir patiently.
2. Make sure you cook the onion until it takes a golden-brown color while the heat is lowered. If the onions start sticking to the pan, use some water to sprinkle on them.
3. Once done, add vinegar to the preparation and mix the contents together. Cook for 40-50 seconds and turn off the heat.
4. Use a bowl to store the contents. Cool completely.
5. Once cool, add some Greek yogurt and whisk well.
6. Serve the dish at room temperature or store and serve chilled with crackers or vegetable sticks.

Bread-less Subs

Serves: 6

Ingredients:

- 12 slices salami
- 2 tbsp. red wine vinegar
- 1/2 cup keto conducive mayonnaise
- 1 cup shredded Romaine lettuce
- 1 tbsp. extra-virgin olive oil
- 4 small clove garlic, grated
- 1 tsp. Italian dressing
- 6 slices ham
- 6 slices provolone cheese
- 1/2 cup roasted red peppers
- 12 slices pepperoni

Directions:

1. Recipe for Italian dressing: Add, garlic, vinegar, oil, mayonnaise and Italian dressing into a bowl and whisk until the mixture is ready and smooth.
2. For assembling the dish: Take a platter and place the ham slices on it. Use four slices of salami and four slices of pepperoni to layer the ham. Use slices of provolone to layer each of them.
3. Take the romaine lettuce, divide it consistently and spread it over the cheese in the middle of the dish.
4. Sprinkle roasted red peppers.
5. Use some Italian dressing and spoon it onto the dish. Make sure each of it is rolled and placed down with the seam side facing downwards.
6. Serve.

Sprout Crisps

Serves: 6

Ingredients:

- 1-pound Brussels sprouts, slice thinly
- Caesar dressing to serve
- 4 tbsp. freshly grated Parmesan cheese + extra to garnish
- 2 tbsp. extra-virgin olive oil
- 2 tsp. garlic powder
- Salt according to taste
- Freshly ground pepper to taste

Directions:

1. Take the sprouts and place in a deep bowl. Use oil to garnish it. Use pepper, Parmesan, salt, and garlic powder and sprinkle over it. Toss all the contents properly.
2. Take a baking sheet and line it with parchment paper. Take out the Brussels sprouts and transfer it on the baking dish. Spread all of it evenly in a single consistent layer.
3. Bake in a preheated oven at 400° F for about 20 minutes or until golden brown and crispy. Turn the Brussels sprouts halfway through baking.
4. Use Parmesan cheese to sprinkle on top.
5. Serve alongside a delicious dressing of Caesar as a dip

Cheesy Tacos

Serves: 20-24 (2 crisps per person)

Ingredients:

- 2 tbsp. shredded Parmesan cheese
- 1 ½ cups finely shredded full-fat sharp cheddar cheese
- ¼ tsp. cayenne pepper or to taste
- 1/8 tsp. ground cumin
- 1/8 tsp. chili powder

Directions:

1. Collect all ingredients into a bowl and proceed to toss.
2. Use a baking sheet and put a silicone baking parchment on top of it.
3. Take tbsp. of the mixed ingredients and place in heaps on the silicone sheet.
4. Make sure the crisps are kept at one inch.
5. Once done, lightly scatter the crisps and apply pressure.
6. Bake in a preheated oven at 400° F for 5 minutes until light golden brown on top.
7. Remove from oven and cool for about 30 seconds. Loosen the crisps with a metal spatula. Cool completely.
8. Serve once this process is complete.
9. Use an airtight container for leftovers.
10. Store at room temperature. It can be preserved for 4-5 days after preparation.

Cinnamon Biscuits

Serves: 16

Ingredients:

- 2 cup almond flour
- 1 tsp. liquid stevia or a pinch stevia powder
- 2 small egg
- 1/2 cup salted butter, normal temperature
- 1 tsp. ground cinnamon
- 1 tsp. vanilla extract

Directions:

1. Collect all the ingredients and mix them in a bowl used for mixing.
2. Separate the mixture into 12-16 equal portions and give it a spherical shape. Place on a greased baking sheet.
3. Every biscuit should have a two-inch gap.
4. Once done, press the biscuits with light touch.
5. Bake in a preheated oven at 300° F for 5 minutes. Remove the baking sheet from the oven and press the biscuits with a fork, to get fork marks on it. Continue baking for another 15-18 minutes or until light golden brown on the edges. Remove from oven and cool for about 5-8 minutes. Loosen the biscuits with a metal spatula. Cool completely and serve.
6. Transfer leftovers into an airtight container. Store at room temperature. It can last for 4-5 days.

Chicken Crisps with Parmesan

Serves: 4

Ingredients:

- 20 frozen wing sections (wings and drums)
- 4 tbsp. garlic infused olive oil
- 2 tsp. garlic powder
- 1 tsp. garlic salt
- 1 cup Parmesan, grated

Directions:

1. Take a baking rack and put the wings on it. Sprinkle garlic salt. Place the rack in the oven. Place a baking pan below it.
2. Preheated oven at 400°F. Proceed to bake it for about 30 minutes in the oven or wait until done.
3. Use some garlic oil to garnish and brush on the chicken wings.
4. Make sure to make the skin crispy. Broil for five minutes for this purpose. Remove from the oven and place in a bowl.
5. Use the leftover garlic oil and pour over it and toss well.
6. Use garlic powder and Parmesan as sprinkles and toss well.
7. Serve immediately for a fun evening snack.

Keto Crackers

Serves: 18

Ingredients:

- ¼ cup ground chia seeds
- ½ cup + 2 tbsp. ice water
- 1 tbsp. husk powder
- 1 tbsp. olive oil
- 1/8 tsp. xanthan gum
- 1/8 tsp. paprika
- 1/8 tsp. pepper
- 1/8 tsp. gum
- 1.5 ounces cheddar cheese, shredded
- 1/8 tsp. garlic powder
- 1/8 tsp. dried oregano
- 1/8 tsp. onion powder
- Salt according to taste

Directions:

1. Keep all the dry ingredients into a bowl and stir methodically.
2. Take some oil, pour and mix until the texture is moist and sand like.
3. Add water and mix to form dough.
4. Mix in the cheddar cheese using your hands.
5. Place the dough on a nonstick baking mat.
6. Roll the dough using a rolling pin until thin.
7. Bake in a preheated oven at 375°F for about 25-30 minutes.
8. Remove the baking sheet from the oven. Cut the preparation into eighteen proportionate squares.
9. Place the baking sheet back in the oven and bake until crisp.
10. Remove from the oven and cool completely.
11. Transfer leftovers into an airtight container.
12. Store at room temperature. It can last for 4-5 days.

Pork and Cheese Pockets

Serves: 6

Ingredients:

- 3 tbsp. almond flour
- 2 slices bacon, cooked
- 1 tbsp. thinly sliced green onion
- 1 cup mozzarella cheese, shredded
- 1 tbsp. feta cheese, crumbled
- 2-3 tsp. mayonnaise
- Salt according to taste
- Pepper according to taste

Directions:

1. Use a nonstick pan and place it on the stove over medium intensity heat.
2. Put almond flour and mozzarella on the pan. Stir the mixture until it takes dough like consistency. Turn off the heat once done.
3. Use a sheet of parchment paper and place the dough on it. Place another sheet of baking paper over it. Roll it using a rolling pin. Use a cookie cutter to split the dough into six rounds.
4. Pick the scrap dough and warm it in the pan again.
5. Repeat step 2 and make more rounds. You should have six rounds in all.
6. Place the rounds in greased muffin tins. Spoon in some onion, feta, and bacon.
7. Bake in a preheated oven at 350°F for 15-20 minutes or until the edges turn brown.
8. Garnish with mayonnaise and serve.

Mushrooms with Stuffing

Serves: 16

Ingredients:

- 24 large Portobello mushrooms, remove the stems
- 12 slices cheese, chopped
- 24 ounces fresh kale, discard hard stems and ribs, chopped
- 8 tbsp. extra virgin olive oil

Directions:

1. Take the mushrooms and place them in stem side facing up position on a baking sheet. Sprinkle oil over the mushrooms.
2. Bake in a preheated oven at 375°F for 10 minutes.
3. Once done, place kale on the mushroom caps and place a slice of cheese on each cap.
4. Bake for 2-3 minutes. Broil for a about a minute and a half.
5. Serve hot and enjoy with your friends.

Fish and Avocado Pops

Serves: 12

Ingredients:

- 1 can tuna, drained
- 1 medium avocado, pitted, cubed, and peeled
- 1/3 cup almond flour and some extra to dredge
- 1/4 tsp. onion powder
- 1/2 tsp. garlic powder
- Salt according to taste
- 1/4 cup mayonnaise
- 1/4 cup grated Parmesan cheese
- 1/2 cup coconut, to fry
- Pepper according to taste

Directions:

1. Add almond flour, garlic powder flour, onion powder, tuna, salt, pepper, mayonnaise and Parmesan cheese into a big bowl for mixing. Keep whisking until all the ingredients are well amalgamated.
2. Take avocado, add it to the mixture and fold gently. Divide the mixture into 12 congruent proportions and shape into balls.
3. Use a non-stick pan and put it on the flame over medium heat. Put oil and heat.
4. The oil should be properly heated but not smoking hot. Once done, add the tuna spheres in batches and cook until it takes a golden-brown color.

Nachos with Bell Peppers and Beef

Serves: 16

Ingredients:

- 8 medium bell peppers (1 in each color), halved, deseeded, cut into sixths
- 1 cup guacamole
- 4 tbsp. vegetable oil
- 1 cup Pico de Galla
- 1 tsp. ground cumin
- 1/2 tsp. dried oregano
- 1-pound ground beef (80/20)
- 4 cups shredded Mexican cheese blend
- 1 tsp. paprika
- 1/2 tsp. pepper powder
- Red pepper flakes according to taste
- 1/2 cup full-fat sour cream
- 1 tsp. chili powder
- 1 tsp. garlic powder
- 1/2 tsp. kosher salt

Directions:

1. Place the bell peppers in a microwave safe bowl. Add salt and water.
2. Cover the bowl and cook on heat set at high temperature for about four minutes. Let the mixture simmer down for 5 minutes.
3. Use some foil to line a sheet used for baking. Take the bell pepper slices and place them with their cut side facing up, next to each other on the baking sheet.
4. Take a nonstick skillet and place it over medium-high heat. Add oil and heat. Add spices and sauté for a few seconds until aromatic.
5. Add beef and salt and stir into the mixture. Cook until brown. Break the mixture at the same time it cooks.
6. Cover the bell pepper pieces with the beef mixture. Garnish with cheese.
7. Before preheating the oven, set it on the mode to broil. Let the mixture broil for a minute.
8. Spread guacamole and Pico de Gallo on top of the beef.
9. Add 1-2 tsp. water into sour cream and mix well. Garnish with sour cream on top and serve.

Tuna and Egg Salad Bowls

Serves: 8

Ingredients:

- 4 large eggs, hard- boiled, peeled, chopped
- 1 tbsp. lemon juice
- 1/4 tsp. grated lemon zest
- 2 can tuna (5 ounces) packed in olive oil
- 6 tbsp. olive oil or avocado oil or mayonnaise
- Salt according to taste
- 4 strips bacon
- 1 stalk celery, thinly sliced
- 16 lettuce leaves
- 2 scallions, sliced
- 2 small tomato, cut into 8 slices
- 2 tbsp. sour cream
- Freshly ground pepper to taste

Directions:

1. Put your stove on medium heat and place a non-stick skillet over it. Add bacon and cook until crisp and golden brown.
2. Remove the cooked bacon with a spoon and place it on a tray lined with paper towels.
3. When the bacon has cooled down, cut it into bite size pieces. Keep some bacon for garnishing the dish later.
4. Add the following ingredients into a bowl; mayonnaise, lemon zest, lemon juice, tuna oil from the can, sour cream, celery, salt and pepper. Whisk them together until everything is properly combined.
5. Fold gently after adding the egg, tuna, scallions and bacon. Taste the mixture and adjust the seasoning if you feel it is necessary.
6. Use salt and pepper for seasoning tomato slices.
7. Bring out a serving platter and place lettuce leaves on it. Segregate the mixed tuna salad among the lettuce leaves. Put a tomato slice in each cup.
8. Garnish with leftover bacon and scallions and serve fresh.

Protein Italian Bites

Serves: 12-16

Ingredients:

For pizza sauce:

- 2 small cloves garlic, minced
- 2 tsp. olive oil
- 2/3 cup canned crushed tomatoes
- Kosher salt according to taste

For keto dough:

- 3 cups shredded whole-milk mozzarella cheese
- 1 1/3 cups almond flour or coconut flour
- 4 tbsp. full-fat sour cream
- Olive oil, to grease
- Salt according to taste
- 4 large eggs, lightly beaten

Directions:

1. Instructions to prepare the sauce: Take all the ingredients mentioned for making the sauce and mix thoroughly. Set the mixture aside for about 30 – 60 minutes. Stir at occasional but consistent intervals.
2. If the oven has multiple racks, place it on the bottom rack. Preheat for fifteen minutes after placing the baking sheet on the rack upside down.
3. Instructions for preparing the dough while oven is preheating: Take a bowl safe for microwaving and put a mixture of cheese and sour cream in it. Cook it on a high flame for a couple of minutes, keep stirring at one-minute intervals until the mixture has combined properly.
4. Make some dough out of salt, eggs and flour; use your hands to bind the mixture together. Take a baking sheet and grease it with oil. Put the dough on the baking paper. Roll the dough into a rectangular shape of about one fourth inch thickness.
5. Remove the baking sheet from the bottom rack and once lifted place the baking sheet carefully on the pizza stone.
6. Bake in a preheated oven at 450°F for ten to fifteen minutes or till the point it is puffed up and golden brown.

7. Remove the baking sheet from the oven. Spread the sauce prepared earlier over the dough. Sprinkle grated mozzarella cheese on top of the dough.
8. Continue the baking process until all the cheese melts. Ga
9. Garnish with oregano, salt and red pepper flakes on top.
10. Cut the pizza into twelve to sixteen proportionate triangles and serve.

Chicken with Pesto and Avocado

Serves: 6

Ingredients:

- 4 tbsp. extra-virgin olive oil + extra to grease
- 3 pounds boneless, skinless chicken breasts, chopped into 1-inch pieces
- 4 tbsp. pine nuts, toasted
- Zest of 1 lemon, grated
- 1 cup loosely packed fresh parsley leaves
- 2 medium ripe avocados, peeled, pitted, chopped
- 1 cup loosely packed fresh basil leaves
- 4 small cloves garlic, crushed, peeled
- 2 tbsp. lemon juice
- Kosher salt according to taste
- Freshly ground pepper according to taste

Directions:

1. Preheat a grill or a grill pan.
2. Take a bowl and add some lemon zest and 1 tbsp. of oil and proceed to stir. Put the chicken in the bowl and use salt and pepper for seasoning. Toss well.
3. Take 6 skewers of about ten to twelve inches each and pierce equal number of pieces of chicken on every skewer.
4. Instructions for avocado pesto: Take the remaining ingredients and put them in a blender. Make sure you keep blending until the mixture has the consistency of smooth cream.
5. Make sure you grill the chicken for about five to seven minutes depending on how much it is cooked. Keep turning the skewers at close intervals.
6. Once done, put the chicken onto separate serving plates. Use a spoon to put avocado pesto on top and serve.

Pizza Puffs

Serves: 6

Ingredients:

- 4 ounces cream cheese
- 14 slices pepperoni, chopped
- 2 tbsp. chopped fresh basil
- 8 black olives, pitted, chopped
- Salt according to taste
- Pepper according to taste

Directions:

1. Put all the ingredients into a bowl except basil, olives and pepperoni pieces. Mix the ingredients well.
2. Divide into 6 equal portions and shape into spherical balls. Once done, put them on a serving platter.
3. Sprinkle olives, basil and pepperoni on top and serve.

Tangy Olives

Serves: 6

Ingredients:

- 4 tbsp. extra-virgin olive oil
- 2 sprig fresh thymes
- 2 small strips of orange zest, peeled with a peeler
- 1 tbsp. orange juice
- 1 tbsp. olives
- 4 small cloves garlic, thinly sliced
- 1 tbsp. lemon juice
- Kosher salt according to taste
- Freshly ground pepper according to taste
- 2 small strips of lemon zest, peeled with a peeler

Directions:

1. Place a saucepan overheat turned to medium temperature. Add oil and heat.
2. Add garlic, red pepper flakes, pepper, thyme, salt, orange and lemon zest. Sauté for about a minute or till the garlic turns light golden brown.
3. Use olives as the next added ingredient and cook for a minute. Remove from heat.
4. Pour lemon juice and orange juice into the mixture and stir.
5. Segregate into different bowls and serve.

Pork and Avocado Bites

Serves: 4

Ingredients:

- 2 avocados, peeled, halved lengthwise, pitted
- 8 slices bacon
- 6 tbsp. shredded cheddar cheese

Directions:

1. Preheat the oven after setting it to broiler mode.
2. Take an avocado half and stuff it with cheese. Cover it with the other avocado half.
3. Take the piece of avocado and place it with 8 slices bacon on a baking sheet lined with foil.
4. Let it stay in the oven for five minutes and broil until it turns brown and crispy.
5. Take it out and invert the avocado again and broil it until crisp.
6. Once done, take it out of the oven and proceed to chop it into pieces. When the dish has cooled down to a bearable temperature, cut into four halves cross wise and serve.

Strawberry Shortcake Fat Bombs

Serves: 6

Ingredients:

- 3 tbsp. almond flour
- 1 tbsp. shredded coconut plus some extra to roll if desired
- 1 tbsp. coconut flour
- 1/4 cup strawberries
- 1/4 tbsp. coconut oil
- 1/4 tsp. vanilla extract
- 1/4 tsp. stevia

Directions:

1. Place almond flour, coconut, coconut flour, vanilla, strawberries, stevia and coconut oil into the food processor bowl and process until well combined.
2. Divide the mixture into six equal portions and shape into little balls.
3. Take the shredded coconut and place it on a plate if you are using one. Dip the balls into shredded coconut and cover evenly.
4. Refrigerate until use and serve.

Pizza Style Bites

Serves: 6

Ingredients:

- 4 ounces cream cheese
- 2 tbsp. fresh basil, chopped
- 14 slices pepperoni, diced
- 2 tbsp. sun dried tomatoes
- 8 black olives, pitted, diced
- Salt according to taste
- Pepper according to taste

Directions:

1. Take all ingredients mentioned other than olives, pepperoni pieces and basil and mix.
2. Separate into six exact portions and shape into balls.
3. Use the olives, pepperoni pieces and basil for garnishing. Sprinkle on top of the balls and serve.

Bacon Wrap

Serves: 12

Ingredients:

- 12 large sea scallops, trimmed, well drained
- 12 large shrimp, raw, peeled, deveined
- 1 tbsp. toasted sesame oil
- 1 lime worth of juice
- 1 lime worth of zest, grated
- 1 tsp. hot red pepper flakes
- 1 tbsp. grill seasoning or coarse salt and pepper
- 4 scallions, very thinly sliced
- 12 slices center-cut smoked bacon, halved

Directions:

1. Use all the ingredients (except bacon) mentioned and add them into a bowl.
2. Use half a slice of bacon to wrap one piece of shrimp. Begin wrapping from the head and end at the tail. Fasten the rolled shrimp and bacon using a toothpick.
3. In the same fashion use one scallop and wrap it completely with one half of bacon slice and tighten it with a toothpick.
4. Keep repeating the previous step and wrap the remaining shrimp and scallops until you have completed the process.
5. Take a slotted broiler pan and place your bacon wrapped shrimps and scallops on it.
6. Bake in a preheated oven at 425°F for 10 -15 minutes until the shrimp takes a pink color and the scallops transforms into a translucent shade.
7. The bacon should be brown and crisp.
8. Serve once ready!

Vegetable Sushi

Serves: 4

Ingredients:

For sushi:

- 2 medium cucumbers, halved cross wise
- 1/2 yellow bell pepper, thinly sliced
- 1/2 red bell pepper, thinly sliced
- 1/4 avocado, peeled, pitted, thinly sliced
- 2 medium carrots, thinly sliced

For dipping sauce:

- 1/3 cup mayonnaise
- 1 tbsp. sriracha sauce
- 1 tsp. soy sauce

Directions:

1. Take out the seeds from the pieces of cucumber. You should have hollow slices of cucumber.
2. Stuff the cucumber slices with the mixture of all the vegetables. Pack them together closely and tightly.
3. Instructions for the dipping sauce: Add all the ingredients for dipping sauce into a bowl and mix well.
4. The sushi must be cut in one-inch thick slices horizontally.
5. Serve to friends and family with dipping sauce.

Cheesy Egg and Ham Rolls

Serves: 8

Ingredients:

- 8 eggs
- 4 tbsp. butter
- 1/4 cup shredded cheese
- 1/4 cup spinach
- 38 slices ham
- 3 tsp. garlic powder
- 2 ½ cups
- 1 ½ cups
- 1/4 cup diced tomatoes
- Freshly ground pepper according to taste
- Salt according to taste

Directions:

1. Set the oven to broil first. Proceed to preheating the oven.
2. Add eggs, salt, garlic powder and pepper into a mixing utensil and whisk properly.
3. Turn the gas to medium heat and place a non-stick pan on it. Add some butter. When the butter melts, add the eggs and stir constantly until the eggs are cooked and scrambled.
4. Mix some cheddar cheese and stir it together. When the cheese melts, add spinach and cubes of tomato and mix properly.
5. Put four slices of ham on your cutting board, slightly overlapping. Use a full tablespoonful of the eggs for heaping over it and spread it proportionately. Roll the mixture and put in a baking dish with the seam side facing down.
6. Continue with the previous step and make the leftover roll ups.
7. Put the baking dish in the oven and broil for 5 minutes or until ham is crunchy and crisp.

Citrus Crab with Avocado

Serves: 4

Ingredients:

- 1/2-pound lump crabmeat
- ¼ cup chopped chives
- 1 tsp. mustard
- 1 ripe avocado, peeled, pitted, chopped into ½ inch chunks
- 1/4 tsp. salt and some extra to season
- White pepper according to taste
- 3 tbsp. lemon juice

Directions:

1. Take a bowl and add avocado in it. On top of it, use one tbsp. of lemon juice and some salt and add. Make four equal portions.
2. All the ingredients left over need to be added in another bowl. Make four separate and proportionate servings.
3. Use a serving plate for placing egg ring on it. Take some portion of the avocado and put it on the egg ring. Press lightly.
4. Take a portion of the crab mixture and place over the avocado and press it firmly. Now tactfully remove the egg ring.
5. Carry out the previous step until you have made the rest of the avocado crab duets.
6. Serve fresh and hot.

Spicy Green Soybean Dip

Serves: 10

Ingredients:

- 4 large cloves garlic, with skin, crushed
- 1/2 tsp. cayenne pepper
- Salt according to taste
- Pepper according to taste
- 4 tbsp. fresh lime juice
- Vegetable sticks akin to celery, cucumber etc. or keto crackers to dip
- 16 ounces shelled edamame beans
- 1/4tsp. ground cumin
- 4 tbsp. olive oil
- 4 tbsp. chopped fresh cilantro

Directions:

1. For this dish, use a skillet and put it on the stove on medium heat. Add garlic and let it cook until it turns brown. Once done, switch off the heat and remove the skin.
2. Add eight cups of water into a saucepan. Put it on medium heat. Once the mixture begins to boil, add edamame beans. Cook for six to seven minutes.
3. Make sure you remove most of the water from it by draining the beans. Keep the water that is left.
4. Use a food processor bowl to keep all the beans in. Add cilantro, salt, oil lime juice, spices, garlic and pulse until well mixed.
5. Use some water and keep adding a tbsp. at every interval and beat till a point it is properly combined and smooth.
6. Pour the dip into a quirky bowl.
7. You can serve this dip with healthy vegetable sticks, keto nachos or keto crackers.

Brownie Keto Bombs

Serves: 4

Ingredients:

- 1/4 cup dark chocolate chips
- 2 ounces block cream cheese, softened
- 1 tbsp. unsweetened cocoa powder
- 1 tbsp. coconut oil

Directions:

1. Take all the ingredients and add them to a blender for mixing.
2. Keep mixing until it is smooth.
3. Make four equal portions of the smooth mixture and shape into balls.
4. Place on a tray lined with baking paper.
5. Freeze until firm and serve after a meal.

Pudding with Almond and Chia Flavor

Serves: 4

Ingredients:

- 2 tbsp. almonds, toasted and crushed
- 1/3 cup chia seeds
- ½ tsp. vanilla
- 4 tbsp. erythritol
- ¼ cup unsweetened cocoa powder
- 2 cups unsweetened almond milk

Directions:

1. Add almond milk, vanilla, sweetener, and cocoa powder into the blender and blend until well combined.
2. Pour blended mixture into the bowl.
3. Add chia seeds and whisk for 1-2 minutes.
4. Pour pudding mixture into the serving bowls and place in fridge for 1-2 hours.
5. Top with crushed almonds and serve.

Chocolate Ice Magic

Serves: 8

Ingredients:

- 2 tsp. vanilla
- 16 drops liquid stevia
- 4 tbsp. unsweetened cocoa powder
- 2 tbsp. almond butter
- 2 cups heavy cream

Directions:

1. Take all the ingredients and add them to a blender for mixing.
2. Keep mixing until it is smooth enough to consume.
3. Place in refrigerator for 30 minutes.
4. Add frosty mixture into the piping bag and pipe in serving glasses.
5. Serve and enjoy with your friends and family!

Serve: 24

Ingredients:

- 4 oz. heavy cream
- 8 oz. cream cheese
- 2 tbsp. erythritol
- 1 ½ tsp. vanilla
- 4 oz. coconut oil

Directions:

1. Take all the ingredients and add them to a blender for mixing.
2. Keep mixing until it is smooth.
3. Pour batter into the mini cupcake liners and place in refrigerator until it sets.
4. Serve and enjoy.

Ice Cream with a Touch of Macha

Serves: 2

Ingredients:

- ½ tsp. vanilla
- 2 tbsp. swerve
- 1 tsp. matcha powder
- 1 cup heavy whipping cream

Directions:

1. Collect all the ingredients. Once done proceed to mix them together in a jar.
2. Seal jar with lid and shake for 4-5 minutes until mixture double.
3. Place in refrigerator for 3-4 hours.
4. Serve chilled and enjoy with your family and friends!

Avocado Ketogenic Brownies

Serves: 4

Ingredients:

- 1 avocado, mashed
- 1 egg
- ½ tsp. baking powder
- 1 tbsp. swerve
- 1/4 cup chocolate chips, melted
- 2 tbsp. coconut oil, melted
- 1/4 cup unsweetened cocoa powder

Directions:

1. Preheat the oven to 325 F.
2. In a mixing bowl, mix all dry ingredients.
3. In another bowl, mix avocado and eggs until well combined.
4. Slowly add dry mixture to the wet along with melted chocolate and coconut oil. Mix well.
5. Pour batter in greased baking pan and bake for 30-35 minutes.
6. Slice and serve chilled/warm.

Very Berry Sorbet

Serves: 2

Ingredients:

- 1 cup raspberries, frozen
- 1 cup blackberries, frozen
- 2 tsp. liquid stevia
- 12 tbsp. water

Directions:

1. Add all ingredients into the blender and blend until smooth.
2. Once you have blended the mixture together, put it in the freezer.
3. Only remove it once it becomes hard.
4. Serve chilled and enjoy.

Pudding with Chia and Raspberry

Serves: 2

Ingredients:

- ¼ tsp. vanilla
- ¾ cup unsweetened almond milk
- 1 tbsp. erythritol
- 2 tbsp. proteins collagen peptides
- ¼ cup chia seeds
- ½ cup raspberries, mashed

Directions:

1. Add all ingredients into the bowl and stir until well combined.
2. Place in refrigerator for overnight.
3. Serve chilled and enjoy.

Chocolate Pudding with a Twist

Serve: 3

Ingredients:

- ½ cup chia seeds
- ½ tsp. vanilla
- 1/3 cup unsweetened cocoa powder
- 1 ½ cups unsweetened coconut milk

Directions:

1. Take all the mentioned ingredients and transfer them to a bowl for mixing.
2. Once done, proceed to mix until it takes a smooth consistency.
3. Place bowl in refrigerator for overnight.
4. Serve chilled and enjoy.

Cocoa Peanut Biscuits

Serves: 24

Ingredients:

- 1 tsp. baking soda
- 2 tsp. vanilla
- 1 tbsp. butter, melted
- 2 eggs
- 1 cup peanut butter
- 2 tbsp. unsweetened cocoa powder
- 2/3 cup erythritol
- 1 1/3 cups almond flour

Directions:

1. Preheat the oven to 350 F.
2. Add all ingredients into the mixing bowl and stir to combine.
3. Make 2-inch balls from mixture and place on greased baking tray and gently press down each ball with fork.
4. Bake in oven for 8-10 minutes.

Cocoa Macaroon

Serves: 20

Ingredients:

- 1 tsp. vanilla
- ¼ cup coconut oil
- 2 eggs
- 1/3 cup unsweetened coconut, shredded
- 1/3 cup erythritol
- ½ tsp. baking powder
- ¼ cup unsweetened cocoa powder
- 3 tbsp. coconut flour
- 1 cup almond flour
- A little pinch of salt

Directions:

1. Take all the mentioned ingredients and transfer them to a bowl for mixing.
2. Once done, proceed to mix until it takes a smooth consistency.
3. Make small balls from mixture and place on greased baking tray.
4. Bake at 350 F for 15-20 minutes.
5. Serve and enjoy.

Mocha Touch Ice-Cream

Serves: 4

Ingredients:

- 1/2 tsp. xanthan gum
- 2 tbsp. instant coffee
- 4 tbsp. unsweetened cocoa powder
- 30 drops liquid stevia
- 4 tbsp. erythritol
- 1/2 cup heavy cream
- 2 cup unsweetened coconut milk

Directions:

1. Take all the mentioned ingredients and transfer them to a bowl for mixing. However, don't add xanthan gum.
2. Once done, proceed to mix until it takes a smooth consistency.
3. Add xanthan gum and blend until mixture is slightly thickened.
4. Once the mixture is ready, proceed to transfer it to the ice cream maker. Keep churning until it takes a thick, palatable consistency.
5. Serve chilled and enjoy.

One Minute Keto Mug Brownie

Serves: 1

Ingredients:

- 2 eggs
- 1 tbsp. heavy cream
- 1 scoop protein powder
- 1 tbsp. erythritol
- ¼ tsp. vanilla

Directions:

1. Add all ingredients into the mug and mix well.
2. Place mug in microwave and microwave for 1 minute.
3. Serve and enjoy.

Protein Peanut Butter Ice Cream

Serve: 2

Ingredients:

- 5 drops liquid stevia
- 2 tbsp. heavy cream
- 2 tbsp. peanut butter
- 2 tbsp. protein powder
- ¾ cup cottage cheese

Directions:

1. Add all ingredients into the blender and blend until smooth.
2. Pour blended mixture into the container and place in refrigerator for 30 minutes.
3. Serve chilled and enjoy.

Sweet Salad for Cheat Day

Serves: 2

Ingredients:

- 1 tsp. erythritol
- 1 tsp. lemon juice
- 1 sage leaf, chopped
- 1 tbsp. blueberries
- ¼ cup strawberries, sliced
- ½ cup raspberries
- ½ cup blackberries

Directions:

1. Add all ingredients into the bowl and toss well.
2. Serve and enjoy.

Little Berry Pops

Serves: 4

Ingredients:

- 1 tsp. liquid stevia
- ½ cup water
- 1 fresh sage leaf
- 1 cup blackberries

Directions:

1. Add all ingredients into the blender and blend until smooth.
2. Pour blended mixture into the ice pop molds and place in freezer for overnight.
3. Serve and enjoy.

Peanut Butter and Avocado Keto Bombs

Serves: 6

Ingredients:

- 1 tbsp. swerve
- 1 avocado, peeled, pitted, and chopped
- 1 cup peanut butter
- 3 tbsp. heavy cream
- ½ cup butter, melted
- ½ cup coconut oil, melted

Directions:

1. Add all ingredients into the blender and blend until smooth.
2. Pour mixture into the mini cupcake liner and place in refrigerator until set.
3. Serve and enjoy.

Cinnamon Almond Balls

Serves: 12

Ingredients:

- 1 tsp. cinnamon
- 3 tbsp. erythritol
- 1 ¼ cup almond flour
- 1 cup peanut butter
- Pinch of salt

Directions:

1. Use all the ingredients and transfer them to the mixing bowl. Once done proceed to mix thoroughly.
2. Cover and place bowl in fridge for thirty minutes.
3. Make small bite size ball from mixture and serve.

Choco Peanut Butter Pops

Serves: 8

Ingredients:

- 1 cup peanut butter powder, unsweetened
- 16 tbsp. cocoa
- 2 cup coconut oil
- 3 tsp. vanilla extract
- 1 1/2 cup shelled hemp seeds
- 1 cup shredded coconut, unsweetened
- 2 tsp. vanilla stevia drops
- 1/2 cup heavy cream

Directions:

1. Pick all the dry ingredients and transfer them to a bowl. Once done, stir it and add some coconut oil and continue stirring.
2. Take a plate and place coconut on top of it.
3. Once done with the previous steps take the rest of the ingredients and mix them with the mixture of dry ingredients.
4. Divide the mixture into eight equal portions and shape into balls. Immerse in the shredded coconut until all sides are coated.
5. Place in the freezer until it sets. Remove from the molds and transfer into an airtight container.
6. Freeze until use and serve!

Lemony Cheesecake with Vanilla Extract

Serves: 4

Ingredients:

- 2 tsp, lemon juice
- 2 eggs
- 1/2 cup of softened cream cheese
- 2 tsp, pure vanilla extract
- 4 tbsp. of heavy cream
- 2 tbsp. erythritol or Stevia

Directions:

1. In a microwave-safe bowl combine all ingredients. Place in a microwave and cook on high for ninety seconds.
2. At every interval of thirty seconds, stir to combine the ingredients well.
3. Transfer mixture to a bowl and refrigerate for at least two hours.
4. Before serving top with whipped cream or coconut powder.

Chocolate Minty Ice Cream

Serves: 6

Ingredients:

- 1 tsp. Peppermint extract
- 2 cups heavy cream
- 1 cup cheese cream
- 2 tsp. vanilla extract
- 2 tsp. Liquid Stevia extract
- 100% Dark Chocolate for topping

Directions:

1. Place ice cream bowl in freezer per ice cream maker instructions. In a metal bowl, put all ingredients except chocolate and whisk well.
2. Put back in freezer for 5 minutes.
3. Pour ice cream into the ice cream maker and churn the ice cream as per the ice cream maker's instruction.
4. Scoop into bowls; top the ice cream with chocolate shavings.
5. Serve.

Rich Almond Butter Cake & Chocolate Sauce

Serves: 12

Ingredients:

- 1 cup almond butter or soaked almonds
- 1/4 cup almond milk, unsweetened
- 1 cup coconut oil
- 2 tsp. liquid Stevia sweetener to taste

Topping:

- Chocolate Sauce
- 4 Tbsp. cocoa powder, unsweetened
- 2 Tbsp. almond butter
- 2 Tbsp. Stevia sweetener

Directions:

1. Melt the coconut oil in room temperature.
2. Add all ingredients in a bowl and blend well until combined.
3. Pour the almond butter mixture into a parchment lined platter.
4. Place in refrigerator for three hours.
5. In a bowl, whisk all topping ingredients together. Pour over the almond cake after it's been set.
6. Cut into cubes and serve.

Ice Cream with Pumpkin and a Touch of Spice

Serves: 12

Ingredients:

- 2 cups of unsweetened almond milk
- 5 tsp. ground cinnamon
- 2 tsp. pure vanilla extract
- 1 tsp. ground ginger
- 2 cups of coconut milk
- 1 tsp. nutmeg
- 2 cups of pumpkin puree
- 1/4 tsp. sea salt

Thickener:

- 1 tsp. guar gum/ 2 tbsp. gelatin dissolved in 1/2 cup boiling water

Directions:

1. Add all the ingredients for ice cream into a blender and blend until smooth.
2. Add guar gum mixture and blend.
3. Pour into an ice cream maker and churn the ice cream as per the manufacturer's instructions.
4. Scoop into bowls and serve.

Peanut-Butter and Coconut Cookies

Serves: 18

Ingredients:

- 2 cups peanut butter
- 1/4 cup Erythritol
- 2 eggs
- 1 1/4 cups coconut flour
- 2 tsp. baking soda
- 2 tsp. peanut extract
- 1/2 tsp. kosher salt

Directions:

1. Preheat oven to 345° F.
2. In a bowl beat the peanut butter, coconut flour and Erythritol with an electric mixer (medium speed) until fluffy. Reduce speed to low and add in the eggs, baking soda, vanilla, and salt.
3. With your hands make balls from the batter and place on parchment-lined baking pan. Leave gap between the cookies.
4. Bake 10 to 15 minutes. When ready, cool slightly and then remove from the oven to cool completely.
5. Serve when it is ready.

Coconut Keto Waffles

Serves: 8

Ingredients:

- 1 cup coconut flour
- 1/2 cup heavy whipping cream
- 5 eggs
- 1/4 tsp. pink salt
- 1/4 tsp. baking soda
- 1/4 cup coconut milk
- 2 tsp. sweetener
- 2 Tbsp. melted coconut oil

Directions:

1. Use an electric hand mixer to beat eggs in a bowl for about thirty seconds.
2. Add the heavy whipping cream and coconut oil into the eggs while you are still mixing.
3. Add the coconut milk, coconut flour, pink salt and baking soda. Mix with the hand mixer for 45 second on low speed. Set aside.
4. Heat up your waffle maker well and make the waffles according to your manufacture's specifications.
5. Serve hot.

Peanut Butter Cake with Chocolate Sauce

Serves: 12

Ingredients:

- 1 cup peanut butter
- 1/4 cup almond milk, unsweetened
- 1 cup coconut oil
- 2 tsp. liquid Stevia sweetener to taste
- Topping: Chocolate Sauce
- 2 Tbsp. coconut oil, melted
- 4 Tbsp. cocoa powder, unsweetened
- 2 Tbsp. Stevia sweetener

Directions:

1. In a microwave bowl mix coconut oil and peanut butter; melt in a microwave for 1-2 minutes.
2. Add this mixture to your blender; take the rest of the ingredients and blend until it is of smooth consistency.
3. Pour the peanut mixture into a parchment lined loaf pan or platter.
4. Leave in the freezer for approximately three hours; the longer, the better.
5. In a bowl, whisk all topping ingredients together. Pour over the peanut candy after it's been set.
6. Cut into cubes and serve when ready!

Chocolate Almond Cake Slices

Serves: 16

Ingredients

- 3 eggs
- 4 oz. dark chocolate, unsweetened
- 1/2 cup coconut oil
- 1 cup almond flour
- 1 cup walnuts
- 2 Tbsp. cocoa, unsweetened
- 1 tsp. vanilla essence
- 2 cups granulated sweetener Stevia or Erythritol
- 1 tsp. baking soda
- Pinch of salt

Directions:

1. Preheat the oven to 350 F.
2. In a container, add almond flour, sweetener, cocoa, salt and baking soda. With an electric mixer, blend the ingredients on the slowest setting until combined well.
3. Melt the chocolate and the coconut oil together (In a microwave or double boiler). Stir thoroughly.
4. Add eggs and vanilla essence to the flour and mix on a medium speed until a thick batter is formed.
5. Add the butter/chocolate mix to the batter continuing medium speed until an even texture is formed. Line a slice tin or square baking tin with wax paper. Fold in walnut pieces then turn the batter into your slice tin.
6. Bake for 25 minutes. When ready let cool on wire rack.
7. Cut into sixteen pieces and serve.

Cookies with Chocolate and Almond Extract

Serves: 12

Ingredients:

- 2 cups almond meal
- 1 1/2 tsp. almond extract
- 4 Tbsp. cocoa powder
- 5 Tbsp. coconut oil, melted
- 2 Tbsp. almond milk
- 4 Tbsp. agave nectar
- 2 tsp. vanilla extract
- 1/8 tsp. baking soda
- 1/8 tsp. salt

Directions:

1. Preheat oven to 340 F degrees.
2. In a deep bowl mix salt, cocoa powder, almond meal and baking soda.
3. Take another bowl and whisk melted coconut oil, almond milk, almond and vanilla extract and maple syrup together. Merge the almond meal mixture with almond milk mixture and mix well.
4. In a greased baking pan pour the batter evenly. Bake for 10-15 minutes.
5. After these steps, let it cool on a wire rack.
6. Proceed to serve.

Instant Coffee Ice Cream

Serves: 2

Ingredients:

- 1 Tbsp. Instant Coffee
- 2 Tbsp. Cocoa Powder
- 1 cup coconut milk
- 1/4 cup heavy cream
- 1/4 tsp. flax seeds
- 2 Tbsp. Erythritol
- 15 drops liquid Nutria

Direction:

1. Add all ingredients except the flax seeds into a container of the immersion blender you need to use.
2. Blend well until all ingredients are incorporated well. Slowly add in flax seeds until a slightly thicker mixture is formed. Add the mixture to your ice cream machine and follow manufacturer's instructions.
3. When ready proceed to serve or store.

Coco Cream with Hazelnut

Serves: 8

Ingredients:

- 2 cups of hazelnut halves
- 4 tbsp. of cocoa powder, unsweetened
- 8 tbsp. granulated stevia (or any sweetener of choice)
- 2 tsp. of non-preservative vanilla extract
- 4 tbsp. of melted coconut oil

Directions

1. Mix all the ingredients properly and put in your blender. Let it blend until it properly smooth.
2. Store the mixture in the refrigerator for about an hour.
3. Serve and enjoy!

Lemon Coconut Pearls

Serves: 8

Ingredients:

- 6 packages of crystallized lemon extracts
- 1/2 cup granulated stevia
- 1/2 cup shredded coconut, unsweetened
- 2 cups cream cheese

Directions:

1. In a bowl, combine cream cheese, lemon and Stevia. Blend well until incorporate.
2. Once the mixture is well combined, put it back in the fridge to harden up a bit.
3. Roll the mixture into thirty balls and immerse each ball into finely shredded coconut.
4. Keep in the freezer for multiple hours.
5. Serve when cool and ready to eat.

Very Berry Smoothie

Serves: 2

Ingredients:

- 1 tsp. vanilla
- 2 tbsp. swerve
- 2 tbsp. cream cheese, softened
- 3/4 cup fresh raspberries
- 4 tbsp. heavy cream
- 1 cup ice

Directions:

1. Take all the ingredients and mix them in a blender until rich, smooth, and creamy.
2. Serve or store in bottle for later consumption.

Energy Enhancing Breakfast Smoothie

Serves: 1

Ingredients:

- 1 cup unsweetened almond milk
- 1/2 cup ice
- 1 tbsp. MCT oil
- 1 1/2 tsp. maca powder
- 1 tbsp. almond butter

Directions:

1. Take all the ingredients and mix them in a blender until rich, smooth, and creamy.
2. Serve to enjoy a hearty breakfast.

Caramel Coffee Smoothie

Serves: 4

Ingredients:

- 1/2 cup almond milk, unsweetened
- 3 tbsp. sugar- free caramel syrup
- 3 tbsp. sugar-free chocolate syrup
- 3/4 cup cold coffee
- 1/2 cup heavy cream
- 2 tbsp. cocoa, unsweetened Ice cubes

Directions:

1. Take all the ingredients and mix them in a blender until rich, smooth, and creamy.
2. Serve or store in bottle for later use.

Blackberry Smoothie

Serves: 2

Ingredients:

- 1 cup unsweetened almond milk
- 1/2 cup ice
- 1/2 tsp. vanilla
- 1 tsp. erythritol
- 2 oz. cream cheese, softened
- 4 tbsp. heavy whipping cream
- 2 oz. fresh blackberries

Directions:

1. Take all the ingredients and mix them in a blender until rich, smooth, and creamy.
2. Serve or store in bottle for later use.

Choco Delight Sunflower Butter Smoothie

Serves: 2

Ingredients:

- 2/3 cup unsweetened coconut milk
- 1/2 cup ice
- 1 tsp. vanilla
- 2 tsp. unsweetened cocoa powder
- 1/3 cup water
- 4 tbsp. sunflower seed butter

Directions:

1. Take all the ingredients and mix them in a blender until rich, smooth, and creamy.
2. Serve or store in bottle for later use.

Cheesy Blueberry Smoothie

Serves: 2

Ingredients:

- 2 cup unsweetened almond milk
- 1 cup ice
- 1/2 tsp. vanilla
- 10 drops liquid stevia
- 2 scoops vanilla protein powder
- 2/3 cup blueberries
- 4 oz. cream cheese

Directions:

1. Take all the ingredients and mix them in a blender until rich, smooth, and creamy.
2. Serve or store in bottle for later use.

Cinnamon Delight Smoothie

Serves: 2

Ingredients:

- 2 tbsp. ground chia seeds
- 1/2 cup vanilla protein powder
- 1 cup water
- 1 tsp. cinnamon
- 1/2 cup ice
- 1 cup unsweetened coconut milk
- 2 tbsp. coconut oil

Directions:

1. Take all the ingredients and mix them in a blender until rich, smooth, and creamy.
2. Serve or store in bottle for later use.

Berry-licious Smoothie

Serves: 8

Ingredients:

- 1 cup blackberries
- 3 cups unsweetened almond milk
- 2 tbsp. heavy cream
- 1 1/3 cup strawberries
- 1 1/3 cup raspberries
- 1 cup unsweetened coconut milk

Directions:

1. Add all ingredients into the blender and blend until smooth.
2. Serve and enjoy.

Avocado Coco Smoothie

Serves: 2

Ingredients:

- 2 cups unsweetened coconut milk
- 2 tsp. chia seeds
- 2 tsp. lime juice
- 10 spinach leaves
- 1 avocado
- 2 tsp. ginger

Directions:

1. Take all the ingredients and mix them in a blender until rich, smooth, and creamy.
2. Serve or store in bottle for later use.

Healthy Veggie Smoothie

Serves: 2

Ingredients:

- 1 cup avocado
- 1/2 lemon, peeled
- 1 cucumber, peeled
- 1 tsp. ginger, peeled
- 1/2 cup cilantro
- 1 cup baby spinach
- 1 cup of water

Directions:

1. Take all the ingredients and mix them in a blender until rich, smooth, and creamy.
2. Serve or store in bottle for later use.

Cinnamon Magic Smoothie

Serves: 2

Ingredients:

- 2 tbsp. shredded coconut
- 1 1/2 cup unsweetened almond milk
- 1 tsp. cinnamon
- 1/2 cup unsweetened coconut milk
- 2 scoops of vanilla protein powder

Directions:

1. Take all the ingredients and mix them in a blender until rich, smooth, and creamy.
2. Serve or store in bottle for later use.

Coconut and Cranberry Smoothie

Serve 1

Ingredients:

- 1 cup unsweetened coconut milk
- 1 tbsp. MCT oil
- 1 tsp. erythritol
- 1/2 cup fresh cranberries

Directions:

1. Take all the ingredients and mix them in a blender until rich, smooth, and creamy.
2. Serve or store in bottle for later use.

Strawberry Blast Avocado Smoothie

Serves: 2

Ingredients:

- 2/3 cup strawberries
- 1/2 cup ice
- 5 drops liquid stevia
- 1 tbsp. lime juice
- 1 1/2 cups unsweetened coconut milk
- 1 avocado

Directions:

1. Take all the ingredients and mix them in a blender until rich, smooth, and creamy.
2. Serve or store in bottle for later use.

Yummy Choco Macadamia Smoothie

Serves: 1

Ingredients:

- 1 tbsp. unsweetened cocoa powder
- 2 tbsp. chia seed
- 1 tbsp. coconut butter
- 1 tsp. MCT oil
- 2 tbsp. macadamia nuts
- 1 cup unsweetened almond milk

Directions:

1. Take all the ingredients and mix them in a blender until rich, smooth, and creamy.
2. Serve or store in bottle for later use.

Ginger Apple Blueberry Smoothie

Serves: 2

Ingredients:

- 1/2 apple
- 1 tsp. MCT oil
- 1/2 tbsp. collagen powder
- 1 tsp. ginger
- 1 cup unsweetened coconut milk
- 1/2 cup coconut yogurt
- 15 blueberries

Directions:

1. Take all the ingredients and mix them in a blender until rich, smooth, and creamy.
2. Serve or store in bottle for later use.

Protein Strawberry Smoothie

Serve 1

Ingredients:

- ☐ 1/3 cup strawberries
- ☐ 1/3 cup water
- ☐ 1/2 cup unsweetened almond milk
- ☐ 1/2 scoop vanilla protein powder
- ☐ 1 tbsp. almond butter

Directions:

1. Take all the ingredients and mix them in a blender until rich, smooth, and creamy.
2. Serve or store in bottle for later use.

Conclusion

After taking a close look at everything involved while following a ketogenic diet, you might have come to draw your own conclusions. Your opinions might be heavily influenced by the different pros and ketones that are associated with ketosis. However, it is very clear that the benefits that are provided by ketogenic diet outweigh its side effects.

Throughout the history of ketogenic dietary practices, we have seen that it has been widely used for treating various diseases such as epilepsy and neurodegenerative diseases since the ancient Greek and Indian civilizations. We have seen how ketogenic diet and fasting were extensively used for reducing the frequency of epileptic seizures in epilepsy patients. There are several medical research studies that exhibit the anti-inflammatory benefits of eating a diet that is low in carbohydrates. After learning how excessive consumption of carbs can cause severe health complications such as chronic inflammation and arthritis, the keto diet seems to be a very good alternative for people who are looking to improve their health and fitness levels.

It is irrefutable that keto diet provides a host of positive health benefits for the body while increasing stamina and endurance at the same time. Have you ever wondered what differentiates an average human being from an endurance athlete or an Inuit capable of lugging 200 pounds across the cold tundra's? It is what they eat that separates these extraordinary individuals from all of us, and as you might have already guessed, their food tends to have a high content of fat instead of pasta and chips. There is enough evidence to support the idea that the keto diet is good for body and health.

Although there might be some side effects when you begin following a ketogenic diet plan, these effects are short-lived and mainly caused as a result of your body adjusting itself to the state of ketogenesis. You can sidestep these side effects by staying hydrated and supplementing your body with enough physical exercise. Keto diet can be useful for achieving several health goals, be it epilepsy management, weight loss, regulation of blood sugar, blood pressure, or reducing inflammation. The good outweighs the bad for ketogenic diet.